Ultrasound and the Endometrium

PROGRESS IN OBSTETRIC
AND GYNECOLOGICAL
SONOGRAPHY SERIES

SERIES EDITOR: ASIM KURJAK

Ultrasound and the Endometrium

Edited by

A. C. FLEISCHER, A. KURJAK and S. GRANBERG

The Parthenon Publishing Group
International Publishers in Medicine, Science & Technology

NEW YORK   LONDON

Library of Congress Cataloging-in-Publication Data

Ultrasound and the endometrium/edited by
A. C. Fleischer, A. Kurjak, and S. Granberg.
    p. cm.—(Progress in obstetric and
gynecological sonography series)
  Includes bibliographical references and index.
  ISBN 1-85070-906-8
  1. Endometrium—Ultrasonic imaging.
  2. Transvaginal ultrasonography.
  3. Endometrium—Diseases—Diagnosis.
I. Fleischer, A. C. II. Kurjak, Asim.
III. Granberg, S. IV. Series.
  [DNLM: 1. Endometrium—ultrasonography.
2. Endometrium—pathology. 3. Ultrasonography—methods. WP 400 U47 1996]
RG316.U48 1996
618.1—dc21
DNLM/DLC
for Library of Congress   97-2669
                                 CIP

British Library Cataloguing in Publication Data

Ultrasound and the endometrium. — (Progress
  in obstetric and gynecological sonography
  series)
  1. Endometrium — Ultrasonic imaging
  2. Endometrium — Diseases — Diagnosis
  3. Transvaginal ultrasonography
  I. Fleischer, A. C. II. Kurjak, Asim
  III. Granberg, S.
  618.1'07543

  ISBN 1-85070-906-8

Published in the USA by
The Parthenon Publishing Group Inc.
One Blue Hill Plaza
Pearl River
New York 10965, USA

Published in the UK and Europe by
The Parthenon Publishing Group Ltd.
Casterton Hall, Carnforth
Lancs. LA6 2LA, UK

Copyright © 1997 Parthenon Publishing Group

First published 1997

Typeset by AMA Graphics Ltd., Preston, UK
Printed and bound in Spain by T. G. Hostench, S.A.

Contents

List of principal contributors

F. Bonilla-Musoles
Departamento Obstetricia y Ginecologia
Facultad de Medicina de Valencia
Hospital Clinico Universitario
Avda. Blasco Ibáñez 17
46010 Valencia
Spain

T. J. Dubinsky
Department of Radiology
University of Texas-Houston,
LBJ General Hospital
5656 Kelley Ave, Houston, TX 77025
USA

C. Exacoustòs
Department of Obstetrics and Gynecology
Università degli Studi di Roma, Tor Vergata
Policlinico S. Eugenio Piazzale
    dell'Umanesimo
00144 Rome
Italy

A. C. Fleischer
Department of Radiology and Radiological
    Sciences
Vanderbilt University Medical Center
CCC-1121 Medical Center North
1161 21st Avenue, South
Nashville, TN 37232-2675
USA

S. Granberg
Department of Obstetrics and Gynecology
University of Göteborg
Sahlgrenska Hospital, S-413 45 Göteborg
Sweden

M. Hirai
Department of Obstetrics and Gynecology
Toyo Hospital
12100 Miyagawa, Hikari-machi
Sousa-gun
Chiba 289-17
Japan

O. Istre
Department of Obstetrics and Gynecology
The Central Hospital of Hedmark County
N-2300 Hamar
Norway

D. Jurkovic
Gynaecological Ultrasound Research Unit
Academic Department of Obstetrics and
    Gynaecology
King's College School of Medicine and
    Dentistry
Denmark Hill
London SE5 8RX, UK

S. Kupesic
Department of Obstetrics and Gynecology
Medical School University of Zagreb
Sveti Duh 64
10000 Zagreb
Croatia

A. Kurjak
Department of Obstetrics and Gynecology
Medical School University of Zagreb
Sveti Duh 64
10000 Zagreb
Croatia

M. Wikland
Department of Obstetrics and Gynecology
University of Göteborg
Sahlgrenska Hospital
S-413 45 Göteborg
Sweden

I. Zalud
Winthrop University Hospital
Department of Obstetrics and Gynecology
259 First Street
Mineola, NY 11501
USA

Foreword

Transvaginal sonography has become an accurate means to assess the endometrium. In fact, it has assumed a pivotal role in the assessment of patients with dysfunctional uterine bleeding, infertility, and those taking hormone replacement or tamoxifen.

This monograph discusses and illustrates these many applications. It also presents information on the sonographic depiction of physiological changes, and, in particular, blood flow to the myometrium and endometrium. The monograph also contains new technological developments such as three-dimensional ultrasonography that may enhance sonographic depiction of the endometrium.

It is hoped that this material will be of use to the ultrasound practitioner as a means to convey the many applications of transvaginal sonography in the evolution of endometrial disorders.

A. C. Fleischer
A. Kurjak
S. Granberg

Transvaginal sonography of the normal endometrium

1

A. C. Fleischer, M. I. Applebaum and A. K. Parsons

INTRODUCTION

Transvaginal sonography affords detailed depiction of the endometrium. In order for one to diagnose an endometrial abnormality, complete and in-depth understanding of the transvaginal sonographic appearance of the normal endometrium is needed[1]. This chapter will describe the morphological appearance (thickness and sonographic texture) of the normal endometrium as it is depicted with transvaginal sonography, as well as its vascularity as shown with transvaginal color Doppler sonography.

SCANNING AND INSTRUMENTATION

To depict the endometrium optimally, it is best to use a high-frequency (greater than 6 MHz) transvaginal probe which has both a short internal focus, and a transducer surface architecture optimal for pelvic imaging and high line density (Figure 1). Because the endometrium has an irregular geometry, it is very important to be aware, first, that measurement errors can occur if the operator does not have a full understanding of the image plane in which the endometrium is depicted (Figures 1 and 2) and, second, if measurements are obtained while a uterine contraction affecting the endometrium is occurring (Figure 3). The endometrium is best depicted on transvaginal sonography in the sagittal plane (Figure 1). In the sagittal plane, the endocervical canal is seen continuing into the endometrial canal. Tilting the angle of the probe or imaging a uterus that is either slightly rotated and/or deviated from the midline may result in overestimation of endometrial thickness. Interobserver measurement error has been estimated[2] to be 1.5 mm.

For most patients who do not have significant amounts of intraluminal fluid, the endometrium is measured in a bilayer thickness from the proximal myometrial–endometrial junction to the distal myometrial–endometrial junction. If intraluminal fluid is present, each endometrial thickness should be measured separately, and the combined endometrial thickness should be expressed as a sum of the two layers (Figure 4).

Measurement errors can occur when the endometrial width, as depicted in the semi-coronal plane, is measured, rather than in the correct sagittal orientation. In this plane, the endometrial invagination in the tubal ostia can be observed, indicating that the image plane is in a coronal, rather than a sagittal, orientation (Figure 4). Short-axis views where the transducer is placed in the mid-vagina and the probe is tilted sharply anteriorly for anteflexed uteri can reveal a short-axis approximation of the bilayer endometrial thickness.

Wave-like endometrial motion resulting from myometrial contractions may result in slight differences in assessment of endometrial thickness (Figures 4h and i). Peristaltic waves can be easily recognized on high-speed playback of videotape and, in some patients, in real-time examinations, as a change in the relative configuration and thickness of the endometrium. These peristaltic waves have a role in sperm transport and during menstruation[3].

One must be aware that endometrial appearance should always be interpreted in the light of follicular or ovarian function and whether or not the patient is on hormone replacement therapy. Accordingly, secretory phase endometrium should be present when there is a

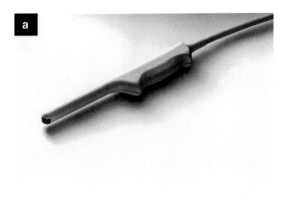

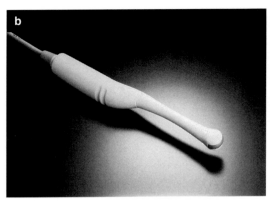

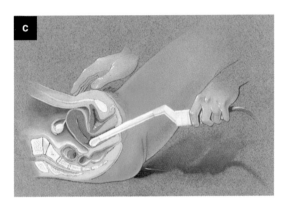

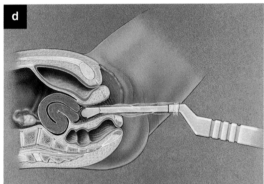

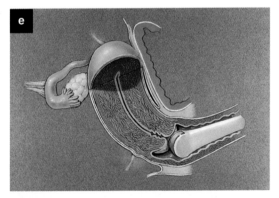

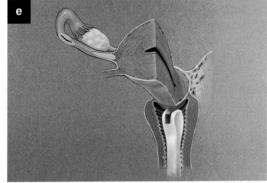

Figure 1 Transvaginal probes and scan planes. (a) ATL's transvaginal probe curved array with frequencies ranging from 9 to 5 MHz; (b) Toshiba's 6 MHz curvilinear TV probe; (c) transvaginal imaging in an anteflexed uterus with the probe directed anteriorly. The free hand can exert pressure better to orient the uterus; (d) similar to (c) but with a retroflexed uterus (the probe should be directed posteriorly for retroflexed uteri); (e) sagittal in side (left) and top (right) views; (f) semicoronal; (g) short axis; (h) combined transvaginal sonography images of endometrium and ovary (a periovulatory endometrium is present, associated with a mature follicle). *Continued on p. 3*

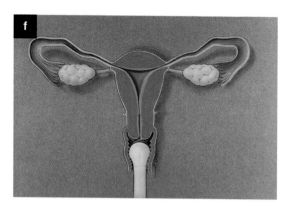

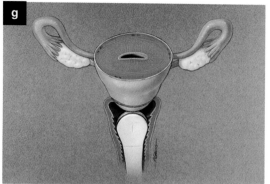

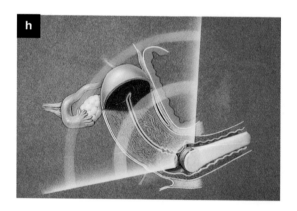

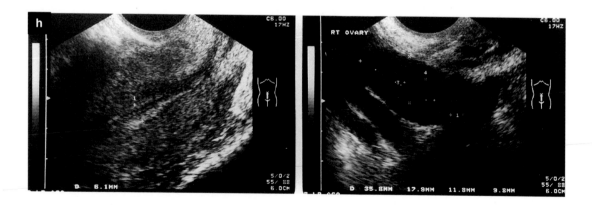

Figure 1 *continued*

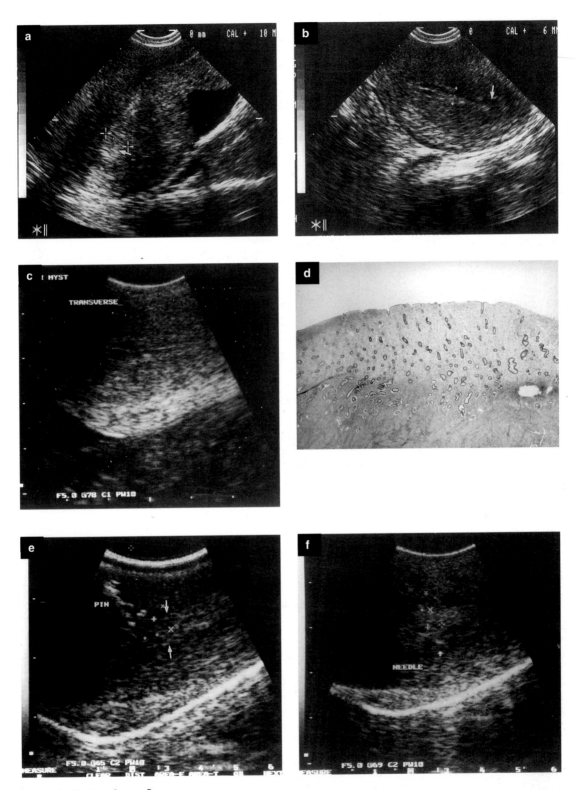

Figure 2 *Continued on p. 5*

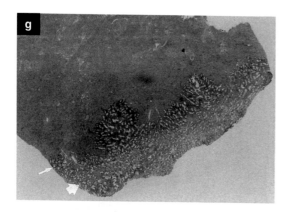

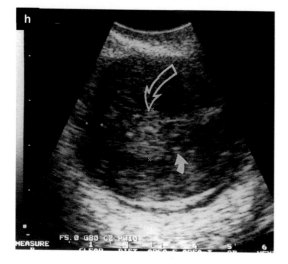

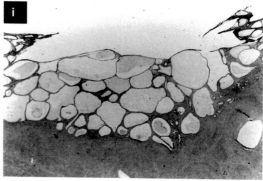

Figure 2 Sonographic–histological correlations. (a,b) *In vivo* transvaginal sonograms showing the difference in appearance of the endometrium when imaged 'down the barrel' (a) versus short axis (b). When imaged 'down the barrel', the interface between glands and stroma is more perpendicular to the beam. There is a 4-mm difference in measurement (between cursors) of the bilayer thickness when imaged in the semicoronal and short axes. The arrows point to the posterior fundal area, which has a different echogenicity dependent on scan plane. (c) *In vitro* sonogram showing multilayered endometrium typical of mid-cycle development. The outer echogenic layer corresponds to the basalis layer, whereas the inner hypoechoic layer represents the functionalis (d). The glandular elements are relatively sparse when compared to the stroma, and the parallel glands are relatively straight and narrow compared to those seen in the secretory phase. (e,f) *In vitro* sonograms showing the area sampled marked with a pin. The endometrium is echogenic in long (e) and short (f) axes. The histological specimen (g) taken at the designated area shows a secretory pattern consisting of numerous distended glands (fat arrow) that become smaller towards the basalis (thin arrow). (h,i) An example of the hyperechoic effect of glandular dilatation and a high gland-to-stroma ratio. This transvaginal sonogram (h) shows increased endometrial echogenicity (open arrow) with scattered foci within the myometrium. Histological examination (i) revealed benign cystic atrophy in both endometrium and surrounding foci of adenomyosis. Thus, any condition which produces glandular dilatation and stromal compression will render endometrium (at any site) hyperechoic

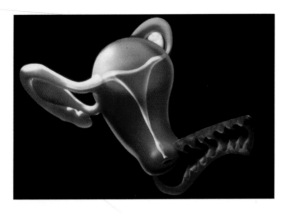

Figure 3 Three-dimensional representation of endometrium (in blue)

sonographically apparent corpus luteum. Conversely, a thin, follicular-phase endometrium should be observed when the ovary is devoid of mature follicles (less than 10–15 mm), and a multilayered endometrium is typically seen when there is a mature (15–20 mm) follicle.

SONOGRAPHIC–HISTOLOGICAL CORRELATIONS

The *in vivo* sonographic appearance of the endometrium correlates closely to the stromal/glandular patterns seen on histological examination[4] (Figure 2). The sonographic appearance of the endometrium is also influenced by the scanning plane in which the endometrium is imaged. For example, Figures 2a and b show the influence of the plane of the scan on the appearance of the endometrium. When imaged 'down the barrel' of the uterus, the endometrium is imaged in its width with the orientation of the glandular elements nearly perpendicular to the beam. When imaged in this plane, the endometrium appears relatively thick and echogenic as compared to its appearance when scanned in short axis.

In vitro comparisons of the sonographic appearance of the endometrium confirm that the texture seen on transvaginal sonography relates to the stromal/glandular composition. Figure 2c is an *in vitro* scan of an excised uterus taken in a waterbath showing a multilayered endometrium with the basal layer as the outermost

echogenic layer surrounding the relatively hypoechoic functionalis. This sonographic pattern can be attributed to the relatively straight and regular orientation of the glandular elements relative to the stroma (Figure 2c). On the other hand, the echogenic texture of the secretory-phase endometrium correlates with enlarged and tortuous glands in the functionalis (Figures 2d, e and f). Other conditions which may produce interfaces resulting in increased echogenicity of the endometrial/myometrial junction interface include cystic hyperplasia of the endometrium and adenomyosis (Figures 2g and h). Much can be learned about the sonographic appearance of the endometrium by comparing the histological composition to the *in vivo* or *in vitro* sonogram.

ENDOMETRIUM IN MENSTRUATING WOMEN

The endometrium undergoes cyclical thickening, denudation and sloughing in normal women of childbearing age. One should keep in mind that the endometrial development is closely correlated to and a reflection of ovarian follicular development and function[5]. Figures 5 and 6 show the range of bilayer endometrial thicknesses in normal women depending on their menstrual status and whether they are pre- or postmenopausal.

The sonographic texture of the endometrium correlates with the presence or absence of a functional layer during the periovulatory period (from 2 days before to 3 days after ovulation) (Figure 4). When there is a functional layer, the endometrium has a multilayered appearance. The echogenic layer corresponds to the basal layer, whereas the hypoechoic layer corresponds to the functional layer. Thus, when there is little or no functional layer, the endometrium is usually echogenic. Stromal edema and high gland-to-stroma ratio present in the secretory phase contribute to the echogenic appearance of the endometrium during the luteal or secretory phase. However, when the endometrium exhibits a multilayered appearance, one can assume that the endometrium has had estrogenic exposure.

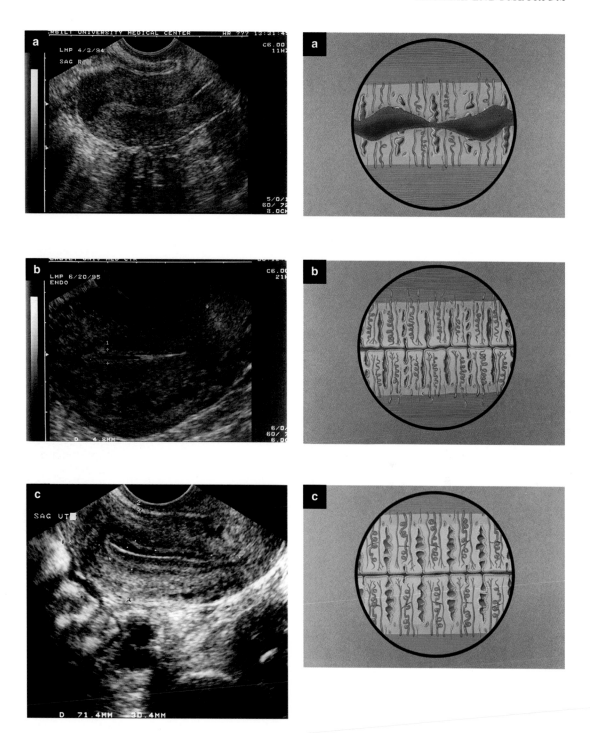

Figure 4 Normal endometrial transvaginal sonograms with accompanying diagrams, depicting the histomorphology of the endometrial layer. (a) Follicular phase; thin, mildly echogenic; (b) periovulatory with trace amount of intraluminal fluid; (c) postovulatory, showing echogenic basal layer and hypoechoic functional layer; (d) luteal-phase endometrium in a retroflexed uterus; (e) luteal-phase endometrium in an anteflexed uterus; (f) luteal-phase endometrium as depicted in a semicoronal plane; and (g) menstrual-phase endometrium as depicted in a short-axis plane. *Continued on p. 8*

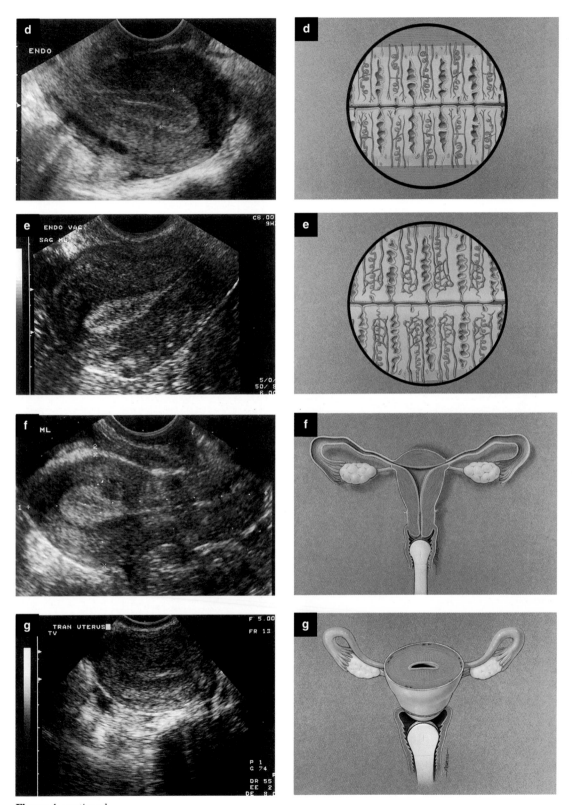

Figure 4 *continued*

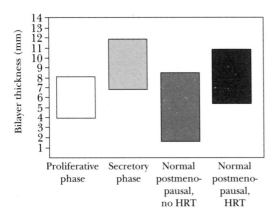

Figure 5 Normal range of transvaginal sonography-measured bilayer endometrial thicknesses. HRT, hormone replacement therapy with estradiol

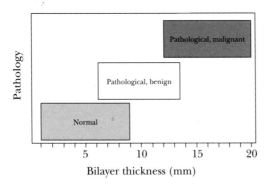

Figure 6 Range of transvaginal sonography-measured endometrial thicknesses in various abnormal groups

In the follicular phase, the endometrium is slightly hypoechoic relative to the myometrium. This is due to its orderly arrangement of straight glandular elements and lack of secretions within and distension of the glands. During the follicular phase, the endometrium usually measures between 2 and 6 mm[6] (Figure 4a).

Prior to the onset of ovulation, the endometrium begins to appear as a layered structure. The outer echogenic layer most likely represents basalis, whereas the hypoechoic internal layer most likely represents the functionalis layer of endometrium (Figure 4b). In the follicular phase, the functionalis layer contains slender and parallel glands, which viewed end-on provide little or no interface. The center echogenic interface is created by refluxed mucus and the

opposition of two smooth surfaces representing the luminal interfaces. This multilayered appearance indicates a periovulatory endometrial development and normal incremental estrogen exposure resulting in orderly gland growth and proliferation. A tiny amount of fluid and/or mucus may be excluded into the lumen within a few days of ovulation.

During the secretory, or luteal phase, when the endometrium differentiates under the influence of progesterone, the endometrium becomes echogenic from the basal layer inward toward the lumen (Figure 4c). This increase in echogenicity results from glandular enlargement and the numerous tortuous glandular elements and their secretions, which proceeds from the basalis to the lumen. Stromal edema that occurs in the early secretory phase also contributes to this increased echogenicity. During this phase, the endometrium can measure from 12 to 14 mm in bilayer thickness (Figure 4c).

When menses is imminent, there is a slight collapse of the functionalis and the endometrium becomes thinner and more irregular in texture (Figure 4d). During menses, sloughing of the endometrium produces an irregular, and progressively less defined, interface. Subendometrial myometrial peristalsis may also be observed, directed from the fundus toward the cervix.

Intraluminal fluid may be observed during ovulation or in some conditions such as vaginosis that are associated with increased vaginal or cervical secretions (Figure 7). Large hydrosalpinges may drain into the cavity during the secretory phase, and outflow obstruction produces hematometra.

ENDOMETRIUM IN POSTMENOPAUSAL WOMEN

The endometrium in postmenopausal women varies according to their weight, years since menopause and the administration of hormone replacement medications[7-9]. In general, the postmenopausal endometrium is atrophic, with a bilayer thickness measuring less than 5 mm (Figure 8). Occasionally, echogenic interfaces

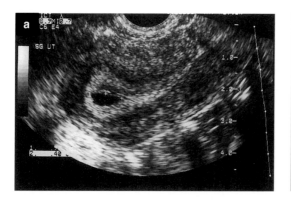

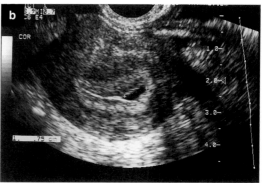

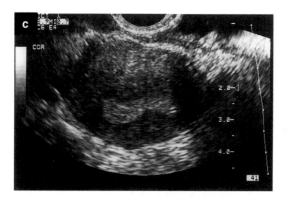

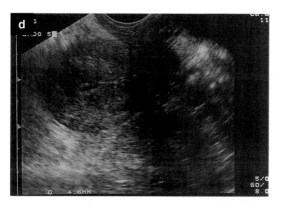

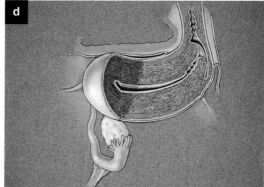

Figure 7 Normal variants. (a,b,c) Intraluminal fluid in a patient with vaginosis as depicted in long (a) and short (b) axes. Two minutes later (c), the fluid was gone. (d) Intraluminal fluid separating normal thin and regular endometrium in a postmenopausal woman. *Continued on pp. 11 and 12*

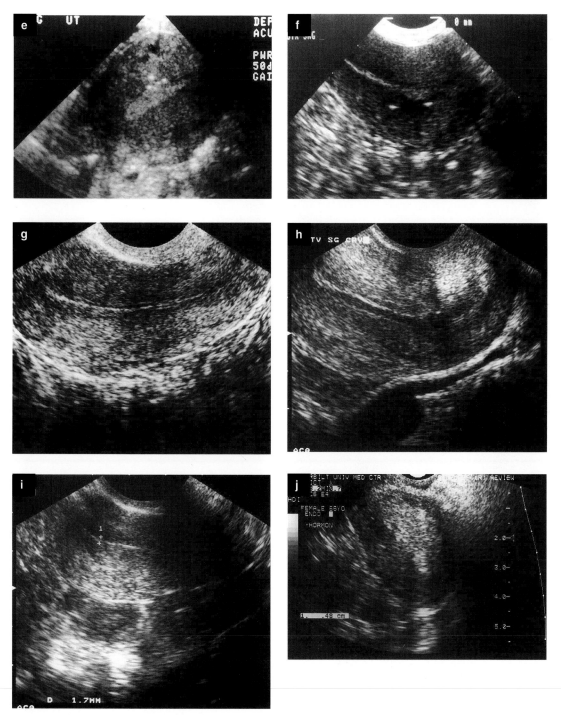

Figure 7 *continued* (e) Echogenic foci within the inner myometrium in a patient with normal endometrial status post dilatation and curettage (courtesy of Mary Warner, MD). (f) Same as (e) in a patient with a thin, normal endometrium whose echogenic foci probably represented fibrotic areas after dilatation and curettage (courtesy of Deland Burks, MD). (g) Thin endometrium in a patient receiving Depo-provera®. (h) Hypo-echoic functionalis layer in the periovulatory period. (i) Thin endometrium (between cursors) in a patient on ovulation suppression. (j) Irregular echogenic myometrium adjacent to normal endometrium. *Continued on p. 12*

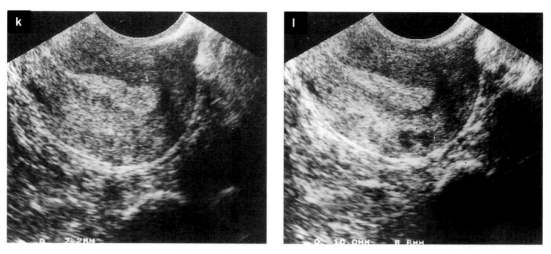

Figure 7 *continued* (k,l) Slight differences in endometrial thickness (between cursors) during and after a myometrial contraction. (l) A small intramural leiomyoma is also seen (between cursors) within the fundus

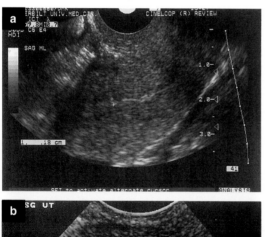

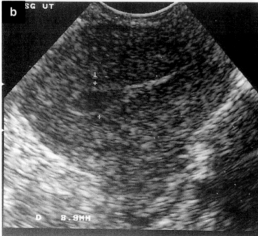

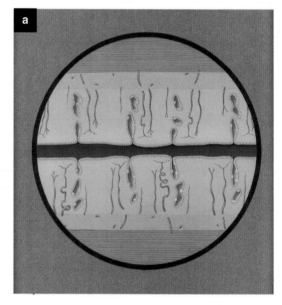

Figure 8 Postmenopausal endometrium. (a) Atrophic (2-mm) endometrium with an accompanying diagram showing sparse glands. (b) Intraluminal fluid separating normal endometrium in a patient receiving hormone replacement therapy

may be seen within the lumen due to trapped mucus or synechiae. More frequently, fluid can be seen within the lumen, but, if the endometrial layers themselves measure less than 4 mm, this is a benign finding.

The effect of hormone replacement treatment on the endometrium depends on the type of medications and their dosage. With unopposed estrogen, the endometrium generally proliferates and almost always measures more than 5 mm. If a combined continuous estrogen–progestin regimen is administered, the endometrium typically measures less than 6 mm, but this may depend on whether the combined treatment is sequential or combined. A cyclic estrogen–progestin regimen produces alternating proliferative and secretory effects that mimic a natural cycle but with maximum thickness of less than or equal to 8 mm.

ANATOMICAL VARIANTS

The endometrium may be used as a guide to evaluate certain uterine malformations, such as bicornuate uteri or septate uteri. In a bicornuate uterus, the endometrium in each uterine horn is best depicted when it is maximally echogenic in the secretory phase. The bicornuate uterus can be differentiated from a septate one in that a fundal cleft is present between the horns.

TRANSVAGINAL COLOR DOPPLER SONOGRAPHY OF THE ENDOMETRIUM

The endometrium is supplied by the radial arteries, which penetrate the myometrium, to give rise to the straight arteries coursing within the basal layer of the endometrium and the spiral arteries which course into the endometrium itself. Flow within these vessels is usually so slow that most frequency-based color Doppler units cannot detect it, and only some authors have recognized it[10]. However, with amplitude Doppler, additional authors have recognized blood flow within the endometrium itself[11,12] (Figure 9).

The blood supply to the endometrium is derived from branches of the uterine arteries. Emanating from the arcuate arteries are the radial arteries. These vessels run through the myometrium to just outside the endometrium, where they form terminal branches of two types: straight and coiled. The straight branches, also known as the basal arteries, supply the basalis layer of the endometrium. The coiled branches, also known as the spiral arteries, traverse the endometrium and supply the functionalis layer. The spiral arteries, like the endometrium and unlike the basal arteries, are responsive to the hormonal changes of the menstrual cycle[13].

In preparation for implantation, around day 22 the endometrium undergoes transformations influenced by increasing progesterone levels. These modifications include: an increase in the rate of blood flow, an increase in the number of cells populating the stroma and epithelium, an increase in uterine oxygen consumption, an increase in oxygen diffusion into the uterine lumen and a generalized transient edema[14].

The spiral arteries respond to the hormonal changes of the menstrual cycle and undergo transformations as well[13]. These responses include: proliferation of the endothelium, thickening of the wall and coiling. These vessels play an important role in implantation. The changes for a normal implantation may be reduced if the spiral arterioles are inadequately developed[15].

Changes in the endometrial vascularity appear present on color Doppler examination, which may reflect the histological changes described by the pathologists[16]. Some investigators appear unable to demonstrate this[17]. Perhaps this is due to differences in equipment and/or technique.

If one divides the endometrial and periendometrial areas into the following four zones:

(1) Zone 1 – a 2-mm-thick area surrounding the hyperechoic outer layer of the endometrium (inner or subendometrial layer of myometrium);

(2) Zone 2 – the hyperechoic outer layer of the endometrium (basalis);

(3) Zone 3 – the hypoechoic inner layer of the endometrium (functionalis); and

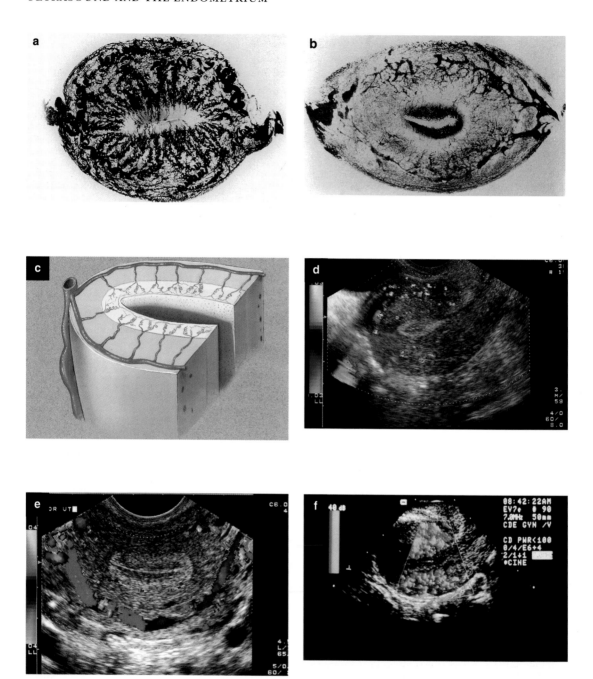

Figure 9 Transvaginal color Doppler sonography (TV-CDS) of the endometrium. (a) Injected and sectioned uterus showing spiral arteries within the endometrium during the luteal phase. (b) Same as (a), showing venous arrangement within the endometrium. Note the greater amount of venous flow when compared to arterial (from Farrer–Brown[18]). (c) Diagram showing arterial supply of the endometrium from the radial arteries which branch into the straight arterioles which course in the basal layer and the coiled arteries that supply the functionalis layer. (d) Frequency TV-CDS showing myometrial flow. (e) Amplitude TV-CDS showing arcuate vessels coursing between the middle and outer layers of myometrium. (f) Amplitude TV-CDS showing vessels within the basal layer of endometrium. (g) Coronal scan with frequency TV-CDS showing flow within zone 3. (h) Same as (f), in the sagittal plane. *Continued on p. 15*

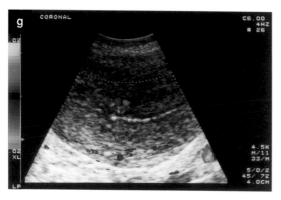 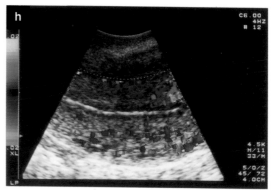

Figure 9 *continued*

(4) Zone 4 – the endometrial cavity (luminal surface);

It is possible to see variations in the depth of vascular penetration before, during and after the mid-cycle (Figures 9f and g). Most patients without diagnosed infertility (presumed normal) usually demonstrate flow into Zone 3 by the mid-cycle[16].

SUMMARY

In summary, transvaginal sonography depicts the endometrium in great detail. Sonographically depictable changes in thickness and texture correlate with microscopic changes. The operator should realize that the endometrium is of irregular geometry and, therefore, is measured best only in a true sagittal reference plan. The texture, as well as the thickness, of the endometrium can be recognized as an indication of endometrial development and hormonal effect and, with the patient's history and ovarian image, can be used as a bioassay. Blood flow can be used as a means to monitor endometrial development.

References

1. Weigel, M., Friese, K., Strittmatter, H.-J. and Melchert, F. (1995). Measuring the thickness – is that all we have to do for sonographic assessment of endometrium in postmenopausal women? *Ultrasound Obstet. Gynecol.*, **6**, 97–102
2. Karlsson, B., Granberg, S., Ridell, B. and Wikland, M. (1994). Endometrial thickness as measured by transvaginal sonography: interobserver variation. *Ultrasound Obstet. Gynecol.*, **4**, 320–5
3. Karl, D., Lyons, E. and Ballard, G. (1990). Contractions of the inner third of the myometrium. *Am. J. Obstet. Gynecol.*, **162**, 679–82
4. Dallenbach-Hellweg, G. (1987). *Histopathology of the Endometrium*, 4th edn, pp. 55–77. (New York: Springer-Verlag)
5. Santolaya-Forgas, J. (1992). Physiology of the menstrual cycle by ultrasonography. *J. Ultrasound Med.*, **11**, 139–42
6. Fleischer, A. C., Gordon, A. N., Entman, S. S. and Kepple, D. M. (1990). Transvaginal sonography (TVS) of the endometrium: current and potential clinical applications. *Crit. Rev. Diagnostic Imaging*, **30**, 85–110
7. Zalud, I., Conway, C., Schulman, H. and Trinca, D. (1993). Endometrial and myometrial thickness and uterine blood flow in postmenopausal women: the influence of hormonal replacement therapy and age. *J. Ultrasound Med.*, **12**, 737–41
8. Nachtigall, M. and Snyder, S. (1990). Endometrial assessment by vaginal ultrasonography before endometrial sampling in patients with postmenopausal bleeding. *Am. J. Obstet. Gynecol.*, **163**, 119–23
9. Granberg, S., Wikland, M., Karlsson, B., Norström, A. and Friberg, L.-G. (1991). Endometrial thickness as measured by endovaginal ultrasono-

graphy for identifying endometrial abnormality. *Am. J. Obstet. Gynecol.*, **164**, 47

10. Applebaum, M. (1993). Ultrasound visualization of endometrial vascularity in normal premenopausal women. In *The Third World Congress of Ultrasound in Obstetrics and Gynecology*, p. 11. (Carnforth, UK: Parthenon Publishing)

11. Applebaum, M. (1995). The menstrual cycle, menopause, ovulation induction and *in vitro* fertilization. In Capel, J. and Reed, K. (eds.) *Doppler Ultrasound in Obstetrics and Gynecology*, pp. 62–71. (New York: Raven Press)

12. Zaidi, J., Campbell, S., Pittrof, R. and Tan, S. L. (1995). Endometrial thickness, morphology, vascular penetration and velocimetry in predicting implantation in an *in vitro* fertilization program. *Ultrasound Obstet. Gynecol.*, **6**, 191–8

13. Dallenbach-Hellweg, G. (1981). *Histopathology of the Endometrium*. (Berlin, New York: Springer-Verlag)

14. Edwards, R. G. (1980). *Conception in the Human Female*. (London, New York: Academic Press)

15. Deligdisch, L. (1991). Endometrial response to hormonal therapy. In Altchek, A. and Deligdisch, L. (eds.) *The Uterus*, pp. 102–14. (Berlin, New York: Springer-Verlag)

16. Applebaum, M. (1993). The 'steel' or 'Teflon' endometrium – ultrasound visualization of endometrial vascularity in IVF patients and outcome. *Ultrasound Obstet. Gynecol.*, **3** (Suppl. 2), abstr. 10

17. Schiller, V. L. and Grant, E. G. (1992). Doppler ultrasonography of the pelvis. In Coleman, B. G. (ed.) *The Radiologic Clinics of North America*, Vol. 30, pp. 735–42. (Philadelphia: W.B. Saunders)

18. Farrer-Brown, G., Beilby, J. O. W. and Tarbit, M. H. (1970). The blood supply of the uterus. *J. Obstet. Gynaecol. Br. Commonw.*, **77(B)**, 673

Endometrial changes as imaged by transvaginal sonography in fertile and infertile women

2

M. Wikland and S. Granberg

INTRODUCTION

Sonography provides non-invasive insight into the changes that occur within the endometrium during the menstrual cycle. Many of the early studies of endometrial changes were performed by abdominal sonography. However, there is no doubt that vaginal sonography is the best way of imaging the endometrium. There are three different sonographic parameters that can be used to evaluate endometrial receptivity in non-stimulated as well as stimulated cycles. These are endometrial thickness, endometrial echo pattern and flow velocity indices as measured by ultrasound.

ENDOMETRIAL THICKNESS

Endometrial thickness should be measured in the longitudinal plane where it seems to be thickest. The measurement should include the hyperechogenic zone surrounding the endometrium (see Figure 1). Ultrasonographic changes in endometrial thickness have been described during the normal menstrual cycle[1–4]. These studies showed a good correlation between increasing endometrial thickness and the characteristic changes of the reproductive hormones in blood. Such correlation with increasing endometrial thickness and steroid levels in blood has also been shown in stimulated cycles[5,6]. Furthermore, ultrasound scanning of the endometrial thickness for prediction of pregnancy in assisted reproduction cycles has been studied by several groups. Rabinowitz and co-workers[7] showed that conceptions did not occur in cycles stimulated with human meno-

pausal gonadotropin (hMG) if the endometrial thickness was less than 13 mm on stimulation day 11. However, they were not able to show any correlation with serum sex hormones and endometrial thickness as measured by ultrasound. In a study by Gonen and co-workers, endometrial growth and the endometrial thickness, as measured by transvaginal sonography the day before oocyte aspiration, correlated with the pregnancy rate in *in vitro* fertilization (IVF) cycles[8]. Despite all the studies published in this field, no real consensus has been reached with

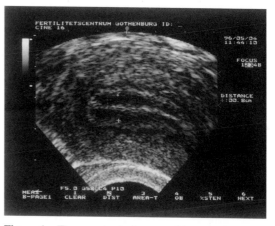

Figure 1 Transvaginal ultrasound image of an anteflexed uterus. The endometrium includes the hyperechogenic zone. The endometrial thickness should be measured in the longitudinal plane at the thickest part. The measurement should include the hyperechogenic zone surrounding the endometrium which most likely represents the basalis layer. Orientation: longitudinal scan with the transducer tip at the bottom of the figure; magnification 1 cm/division on the scale at the left side of the image

regard to the ideal endometrial thickness for an optimal chance of implantation in both non-stimulated and stimulated cycles[9] indicating that the endometrial thickness as measured by ultrasound cannot be used as the sole parameter for predicting implantation. However, an endometrial thickness of less than 7 mm at the time for ovulation or induction of ovulation seems to be not favorable for implantation.

ENDOMETRIAL ECHO PATTERN

It was soon realized that ultrasound was an excellent tool for the characterization of changes in the echo pattern of the endometrium in both natural and stimulated cycles[1,10]. In these early studies, abdominal sonography was used but the full bladder technique was a prerequisite for scanning of the uterus. However, this technique often compressed the uterine cavity and the endometrium, making it difficult to obtain an optimal image of the endometrium. With the introduction of vaginal sonography, it was possible for the first time to examine endometrial changes during the menstrual cycle without any disturbing pressure from a full urinary bladder. Several studies independently showed that three different echo patterns could be distinguished in the follicular phase in both natural and stimulated cycles. Fleischer and co-workers were the first to show that the endometrium gradually increases in reflectivity from hypoechoic to hyperechoic during the cycle. This seemed to be related to increasing tortuosity of endometrial glands, mucin storage and secretion, which thus altered the reflectance of the endometrium. On the other hand, in stimulated cycles there seems to be no correlation between the sonographic appearance of the endometrium and histopathological characterization of the endometrium[12]. However, there is a correlation between the number of endometrial glands as studied by morphometry and the ultrasound appearance[12].

Regarding stimulated cycles, several groups have published data indicating differences in implantation rate with different echo patterns of the endometrium either on the day of human chorionic gonadotropin (hCG) administration or on the day before oocyte retrieval in IVF cycles[3,13–15].

There are three main types of endometrial echo patterns that can be found in all studies published up to date[13]: the hypoechogenic (Figure 2), the triple-line pattern (Figure 3) and the hyperechogenic (Figure 4).

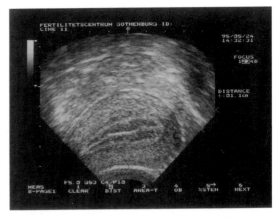

Figure 2 Anteflexed uterus as imaged by transvaginal ultrasound illustrating the hypoechogenic endometrium. The endometrial functionalis is less echogenic (darker) than the surrounding basalis. The typical 'triple-line' endometrial pattern can be seen. This endometrial pattern is typical for the mid-cycle endometrium. Orientation and magnification as for Figure 1

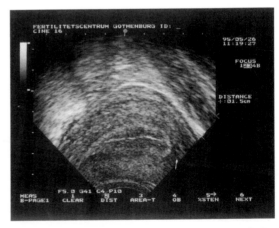

Figure 3 Transvaginal ultrasound image of the endometrium at the time around ovulation or late proliferative phase. Note that the endometrium still has the triple-line texture but the echo pattern is more isoechogenic compared to the myometrium. Orientation and magnification the same as for Figure 1

In order to evaluate the endometrial echo pattern on the day of ovum pick-up in women stimulated for IVF, the endometrium in 127 women was scanned on the day of hCG administration and on the day of ovum pick-up[16]. In all women, pituitary down-regulation was achieved with the gonadotropin releasing hormone agonist nafarelin acetate (Synarela, Syntex AB, Södertälje, Sweden), 0.2 mg administered as a nasal spray twice a day for 2 weeks. For ovarian superovulation, hMG, 225 IU, (Pergonal, Serono Svenska AB, Solentuna, Sweden) was given daily until at least two follicles had reached a mean diameter of 18 mm as measured by ultrasound. Endometrium characterized as triple-line and isoechogenic (Figure 3) on the day of hCG or ovum pick-up resulted in the highest pregnancy rate, 40% (11/28) and 53% (29/55), respectively. In this study, no correlation was found between the endometrial thickness and pregnancy rate if the endometrium had a thickness of more than 7 mm. Our data, as well as those from other studies, clearly indicate that the endometrium has to be thicker than 7 mm and show a triple-line pattern in order to achieve a good implantation rate. There is no doubt that measuring the thickness as well as characterizing the endometrium can

be used for prediction of the probability of implantation. However, further studies have to be performed to determine if the different echo patterns really say anything about endometrial receptivity. If so, ultrasound scanning of the endometrium will be a valuable instrument to establish the optimal time for embryo transfer.

The hyperechogenic zone

Another interesting echo pattern that seems to indicate something about endometrial receptivity is the hyperechogenic zone that surrounds the endometrium (Figure 5). The thickness of this zone seems to vary in stimulated cycles as compared to non-stimulated cycles. When we compare those in our assisted reproduction program with a hyperechogenic zone thicker than 2 mm with those with a zone less than 2 mm (Figures 6 and 7) at the day for hCG injection, there were significantly more pregnancies in the group where the hyperechogenic zone was less than 2 mm (35% versus 10%). It was also found that, in women receiving frozen–thawed pre-embryos in non-stimulated cycles, a hyperechogenic zone of > 2 mm was more frequent in women with unexplained infertility and with polycystic ovarian syndrome-like ovaries as

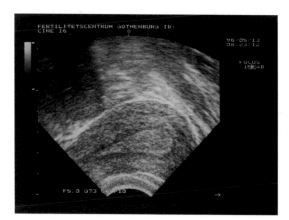

Figure 4 Transvaginal ultrasound image of the endometrium at the time of the luteal phase illustrating the echocharacteristic of the secretory endometrium. In the luteal phase, the echo becomes hyperechogenic compared to the myometrium. The triple-line texture usually disappears. Orientation and magnification as in Figure 1

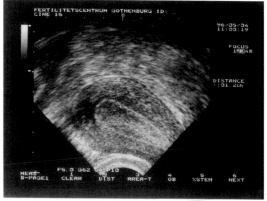

Figure 5 Retroflexed uterus as imaged by vaginal ultrasound with the endometrium surrounded by a hyperechogenic zone seen as a distinct white line. Day 14 in a gonadotropin-stimulated cycle. Orientation and magnification as in Figure 1

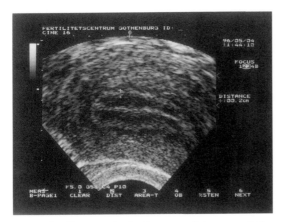

Figure 6 Transvaginal ultrasound image of the uterus on day 13 in a gonadotropin-stimulated cycle. Note the thickness (2 mm) of the hyperechogenic zone as measured between the two white crosses seen on the upper white line. Orientation and magnification as in Figure 1

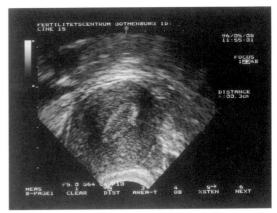

Figure 7 Transvaginal image of the uterus and a thick (4 mm) hyperechogenic zone on stimulation day 13 in a gonadotropin-stimulated cycle. Measurement between the two white crosses on the right part of the white line surrounding the endometrium. Orientation and magnification as for Figure 1

compared to women with tubal infertility (32% versus 13%). These results indicate that, at the time of the luteinizing hormone (LH) surge, the thickness of the hyperechogenic zone surrounding the endometrium reflects a process within the endometrium that can be negative for implantation.

UTERINE BLOOD FLOW

By means of transvaginal color Doppler, it has been demonstrated that there is a complex relationship between the concentration of ovarian sex hormones in peripheral venous plasma and uterine artery blood flow[17,18]. Steer and co-workers could show daily mean changes in pulsatility index within the uterine arteries correlated to the mean concentration of plasma estradiol and progesterone[18]. Available data suggest an increase in the perfusion of the uterus during the course of the menstrual cycle. It has been shown that the lowest blood flow impedance occurs around the time of peak luteal function, that is, the time when implantation is most likely to occur. By means of transvaginal color Doppler, Goswamy and co-workers have found some evi-

dence that decreased uterine perfusion may be associated with infertility[19]. Furthermore, the studies by Steer and colleagues indicate that measurement of uterine blood flow with transvaginal color Doppler can be used for prediction of endometrial receptivity in assisted conception[20]. In that study, it was found that women who did not become pregnant had a significantly raised impedance to blood flow in their uterine arteries. Furthermore, there was zero implantation if the mean uterine artery pulsatility index was greater than 3.0. These data may have clinical implications in assisted conception cycles. Women with poor uterine perfusion on the day of embryo transfer can then be advised to have their embryos frozen and transferred in a non-stimulated cycle that might be more favorable for implantation.

The data published on transvaginal color Doppler and uterine and ovarian function in non-stimulated as well as stimulated cycles are interesting and have clearly shown that the technique is a useful non-invasive tool for detailed studies of ovarian and uterine physiology. The clinical value of this technique in the diagnosis of infertility as well as in assisted reproduction cycles has to be further evaluated.

References

1. Hackeloer, B. J. (1984). Ultrasound scanning of the ovarian cycle. *J. In Vitro Fertil. Embryo Transfer*, **1**, 217–20

2. Sakamoto, C. and Nakano, H. (1982). The echogenic endometrium and alterations during menstrual cycle. *Int. J. Gynaecol. Obstet.*, **20**, 255–9

3. Randall, J. M., Fisk, N. M., McTavish, A. and Tempelton, A. A. (1989). Transvaginal ultrasonic assessment of endometrial growth in spontaneous and hyperstimulated menstrual cycles. *Br. J. Obstet. Gynaecol.*, **96**, 954–9

4. Fleischer, A., Kalemeris, G. and Entman, S. (1986). Sonographic depiction of the endometrium during normal cycles. *J. Ultrasound Med. Biol.*, **12**, 271–7

5. Giorlandino, C., Gleicher, N., Nanni, C., Vizzone, A., Gentilli, P. and Taramanni, C. (1987). The sonographic picture of the endometrium during *in vitro* fertilization cycles. *Fertil. Steril.*, **47**, 508–11

6. Shoham, Z., Di Carlo, C., Patel, A., Conway, G. S. and Jacobs, H. S. (1991). Is it possible to run a successful ovulation induction program based solely on ultrasound monitoring? The importance of endometrial measurements. *Fertil. Steril.*, **56**, 836–41

7. Rabinowitz, R., Laufer, N., Lewin, A., Navot, D., Bar, I., Margaliot, E. J. and Schenker, J. J. (1986). The value of ultrasonographic endometrial measurement in the prediction of pregnancy following *in vitro* fertilization. *Fertil. Steril.*, **45**, 824–8

8. Gonen, Y., Casper, R. F., Jacobsson, W. and Blankier, J. (1989). Endometrial thickness and growth during ovarian stimulation: a possible predictor of implantation in *in vitro* fertilization. *Fertil. Steril.*, **52**, 446–50

9. Li, T.-C., Nuttall, L., Klentzeris, L. and Cook, I. D. (1992). How well does ultrasonographic measurement of endometrial thickness predict results of histological dating? *Hum. Reprod.*, **7**, 1–5

10. Smith, B., Porter, R., Ahuja, K. and Craft, I. (1984). Ultrasonic assessment of endometrial changes in stimulated cycles in an *in vitro* fertilization and embryo transfer programme. *J. In Vitro Fertil. Embryo Transfer*, **1**, 233–8

11. Fleischer, A. C., Kalemeris, G., Machin, J. E., Entmann, S. S. and James, E. A. (1986). Sonographic depiction of normal and abnormal endometrium with histopathologic correlation. *J. Ultrasound Med. Biol.*, **5**, 445–52

12. Rogers, P. A. W., Polson, D., Murphy, C. R., Hosie, M., Susil, B. and Leoni, B. (1991). Correlation of endometrial histology, morphometry, and ultrasound appearance after different stimulation protocols for *in vitro* fertilization. *Fertil. Steril.*, **55**, 583–7

13. Welker, B. G., Gemburch, U., Diedrich, K., Al-Hasani, S. and Krebs, D. (1989). Transvaginal sonography of the endometrium during ovum pickup in stimulated cycles for *in vitro* fertilization. *J. Ultrasound Med.*, **8**, 549–53

14. Gonen, Y. and Casper, R. F. (1990). Prediction of implantation by sonographic appearance of the endometrium during controlled ovarian stimulation for *in vitro* fertilization (IVF). *J. In Vitro Fertil. Embryo Transfer*, **1**, 146–52

15. Fleischer, A. C., Herbert, C. M., Sacks, G. A., Wentz, A. C., Entman, S. S. and James, A. E. (1986). Sonography of the endometrium during conception and non conception cycles of *in vitro* fertilization and embryo transfer. *Fertil. Steril.*, **46**, 442–7

16. Wikland, M., Attebo, B., Granberg, M. and Holmgren, E. (1991). Echocharacteristic of the endometrium a possible parameter for prediction of uterine receptivity. Abstracts of the 7th World Congress on *In Vitro* Fertilization and Assisted Procreations, Paris, 115, p. 147. *Hum. Reprod.*

17. Scholtes, M. C. W., Wladimiroff, J. W., van Rijen, H. J. M. and Hop, W. C. (1989). Uterine and ovarian velocity waveforms in the normal menstrual cycle: a transvaginal Doppler study. *Fertil. Steril.*, **52**, 981–5

18. Steer, C. V., Campbell, S., Pampliglione, J. S., Kingsland, C. R., Mason, B. A. and Collins, W. P. (1990). Transvaginal colour flow imaging of the uterine arteries during the ovarian and menstrual cycles. *Hum. Reprod.*, **5**, 391–5

19. Goswamy, R. K., Williams, G. and Steptoe, P. C. (1988). Decreased uterine perfusion – a cause of infertility. *Hum. Reprod.*, **5**, 955–99

20. Steer, C. V., Campbell, S., Tan, S. L., Cryford, T., Mills, C., Mason, B. A. and Collins, W. P. (1992). The use of transvaginal color flow imaging after *in vitro* fertilization to identify optimum uterine conditions before embryo transfer. *Fertil. Steril.*, **57**, 372–6

Transvaginal ultrasound, hormone replacement therapy and management of the endometrium

3

H. Schulman and I. Zalud

INTRODUCTION

About a decade ago, physicians began to encourage postmenopausal women to take estrogen as prophylaxis against osteoporosis, and progestins as prophylaxis against endometrial cancer. It was generally accepted that prescribing hormone therapy had one major drawback, namely increasing the risk of endometrial carcinoma. There still is no agreed protocol for management of the endometrial bleeding when hormones are prescribed, although unexpected bleeding happens in at least 30% of women. There are no data on what is an acceptable biopsy or intervention rate in the management of these problems. There is incomplete knowledge of the effect of hormones on the postmenopausal endometrium.

Most of our understanding of the effect of hormones on the postmenopausal endomentrium is indirect and based upon blind biopsies. This type of data suffers from sampling errors, sporadic time intervals and an absence of topographical analyses of the uterus.

Within the past 5 years, there have been many publications from around the world that have described the endometrial cavity with the aid of transvaginal ultrasound. Most of these studies have been of episodic nature, namely done in the presence of bleeding and before a biopsy. The results of these studies show that there is broad agreement that an endometrial malignancy is present when there is endometrial thickening, and that a thin endometrium has a high specificity against cancer[1–25].

This chapter critically reviews the pertinent literature, and describes a personal experience with transvaginal ultrasound used before and during the management of hormone replacement therapy. The objectives of management were to maintain a thin endometrium, encourage patient compliance, define an appropriate biopsy rate and diminish or eliminate unexpected bleeding.

PATHOPHYSIOLOGY OF ENDOMETRIAL CANCER

Endometrial adenocarcinoma can arise as a focal lesion, a diffuse process, or as part of an endometrial polyp. Most of the available data are from deductive reasoning from uterine specimens, because there has been no opportunity to observe the development of these lesions directly. There is consensus that endometrial hyperplasia may be a precursor to some cancers, particularly those of the diffuse type. The diagnosis of endometrial hyperplasia is complex. Current classifications attempt to differentiate six types, with one, called 'atypical', allegedly the most serious[26,27]. Studies suggest that 10–20% of 'atypical' hyperplasias may progress to cancer. It is not too sceptical to conclude that a group of expert pathologists would not show broad agreement on a series of endometrial biopsies with varying degrees of hyperplasia.

A number of recent studies have investigated cell biological growth factors, receptors and antigens in endometrial cells to identify better the premalignant cell[28]. Estrogen and progesterone receptors increase when there is hyperplasia, but malignant tissues have fewer than proliferative or hyperplastic tissue. There are changes, but as yet they do not provide precise differentiation or prediction. Although these studies are important to our understanding of cancer, they are far removed from clinical reality. In most clinical circumstances, a lesion is found and biopsied. Cervical cytology is unique as a screening tool because it helps to detect a microscopic lesion. Gynecologists seem to have the same hope for biopsy or dilatation and curettage when the screening alert is bleeding.

PREVALENCE OF ENDOMETRIAL CANCER

The risk of endometrial cancer in the lifetime of a woman from the USA is 1 in 45. The prevalence rate of endometrial cancer is around three per 1000. The peak age of occurrence is 59 years. Meta-analysis data suggest a relative risk for endometrial cancer in hormone users of 2.3, and after 9 years it may be as high as 9.5.

Some have argued against routine screening for endometrial cancer because 70% of women present with stage I disease. Surely more work needs to be done, but data have already emerged showing that endometrial cancer detected by ultrasound has more stage I, and better prognostic factors than those whose primary presentation was bleeding[29]. The two largest studies on screening of endometrial cancer using ultrasound in asymptomatic women gave comparable data: cancer in approximately three per 1000, hyperplasia in about five per 1000 and polyps in about five per 1000[30,31]. Dubinsky and co-workers suggested more frequent usage of hysterosonography for preoperative evaluation of thickened endometrium to identify polyps, and insuring adequate tissue sampling to reduce false negatives[32]. An important new question is whether asymptomatic endometrial polyps should be excised.

American College of Obstetrics and Gynecology publications still refer to advocates of baseline, yearly or random biopsy, even though the risk of cancer is only three per 1000 and there are no data supporting efficacy. The same is true of tamoxifen[33,34].

PROGESTINS

Most gynecologists believe that progestins protect against endometrial cancer. However, meta-analysis data *did not confirm* this belief[35,36]. One cohort study suggested decreased risk with progestins, relative risk (RR) = 0.4, but a case–control study suggested increased risk, RR = 1.8. Grady and colleagues concluded that 'Data regarding the risk for endometrial cancer among estrogen plus progestin users are limited and conflicting'[35]. *In vitro* studies suggest that progestins do slow the replication of endometrial cells, but paradoxically stimulate the growth of breast glandular cells[37]. The potential clinical consequences of this are still uncertain.

Multiple biopsy studies have suggested that progestins reverse endometrial hyperplasia, but do progestins prevent cancer? Estrogen given alone creates endometrial hyperplasia. However, most endometrial hyperplasias are not precancerous; there must be 'atypical' hyperplasia to demonstrate the relationship. Woodruff and co-workers showed that, when biopsy is done during treatment with conjugated estrogen alone, there was a 20% incidence of hyperplasia after 1 year. When hormone therapy was stopped, the hyperplasia disappeared[38]. The recent PEPI (postmenopausal estrogen/progestin interventions) study in the USA gave similar findings, namely that estrogen-induced hyperplasia disappears in at least 94% of the cases[39]. An alternative conclusion to the 'estrogen creates hyperplasia' hypothesis is that '*estrogen produces a drug effect that mimics hyperplasia*'. Endometrial diagnoses are not reliable in the presence of hormones.

A NEW APPROACH TO HORMONE REPLACEMENT THERAPY USING ULTRASOUND AND ESTROGEN ALONE

Three years ago the senior author began a study in a private office setting, using ultrasound as the foundation of the management of the endometrium in women on HRT (H. Schulman, unpublished data). Each woman had a baseline transvaginal ultrasound measurement of the endometrial thickness, and hormone therapy was prescribed to maintain an endometrial thickness < 9 mm. When thickened endometrium and unexpected bleeding arose, hormone therapy was withdrawn for at least 3 weeks. If there was persistent thickening, a biopsy was performed.

One hundred and nineteen women were managed. This was inclusive of all women seen during this time period. There were 12 women who did not return for care. The average age of the entire group was 57.6 ± 7.7 years, range 43–80 years. Average parity was 2.2 ± 1.4, range 0–6 (Table 1).

Baseline endometrial thickness in women already on therapy was 4.6 ± 3 mm, range 0–14 mm, median 4 mm. At the time of follow-up the average thickness was unchanged, but the range of change was − 9 to 17 mm. The majority of cases showed little change, but in five cases the endometrium thickened slightly. An increase of 17 mm happened in a 51-year-old, para 4, originally taking sequential conjugated estrogen 0.625 mg and 10 mg medroxyprogesterone, changed to conjugated estrogen 0.625 mg. The change was made because she had generalized symptoms of hormone overdosage. She eventually came to a biopsy because of difficulty in controlling endometrial growth and bleeding. The endometrium was benign. She is now on combination therapy but still bleeding.

Seventy-eight women were placed on hormone replacement therapy for the first time. The therapy recommended was estrogen only, in all but seven women. Baseline endometrium was 2.3 ± 0.8 mm, range 0–5 mm. After therapy it was 4.4 ± 3.2 mm, $p = < 0.001$, range 1–16 mm, median 4 mm. There were six cases (6.8%) where thickness at follow-up was > 8 mm, range 9–16 mm. There were significantly more women with a thickness > 6 mm in the patients receiving progestins.

Forty-seven women reported unexpected bleeding. Fifteen came from those who had already been on medication (37%), and 32 of those newly placed on therapy (41%). Management in most cases consisted of rescanning. If the endometrial echo was < 6 mm, therapy was stopped for 1 week, and then resumed. If the endometrium was more than 8 mm in the 1st year, medication was stopped for 1 week and a new regimen was initiated. Progestins were added in four cases, and, in two, drugs were stopped at the patient's request.

There were six (5%) women (on hormone replacement therapy for more than 1 year) who had endometrial biopsies because of bleeding, and inadequate shrinkage of endometrium after withdrawal of therapy for 3–14 weeks, average 9 weeks. All biopsies were benign except a 63-year-old woman who had an endometrial adenocarcinoma. She had been on sequential therapy for 12 years, and had had two negative

Table 1 Patient characteristics and results

	No previous HRT (n = 78)		On HRT (n = 41)	
Treatment				
estrogen only	71	(91%)**	6	(15%)
combined	4	(5%)	4	(10%)
sequential	3	(4%)**	31	(75%)
Unexpected bleeding	32	(41%)	15	(37%)
Endometrium > 8 mm	2	(3%)*	6	(15%)
Endometrium > 6 < 8 mm	7	(9%)*	7	(17%)
Biopsy	2	(3%)	4	(10%)
cancer	0		1	
Success of estrogen only	68/71			

*$p < 0.05$ for endometrium > 6 mm; **$p < 0.01$;
HRT, hormone replacement therapy

biopsies for bleeding by another doctor in the previous year. Her endometrial thickness after hormone withdrawal for 9 weeks was only 4.3 mm but it was localized (Figure 1).

This is a biopsy rate of 5%, for which there are no comparable data. The optimum waiting time before a biopsy is done needs investigation[45]. A biopsy rate of 5% translates to 50/1000 or a biopsy to cancer rate of 16/1000 comparable to cervix and breast.

The data presented in this study have the limitations of a private practice environment. It is a feasibility study, to test the hypothesis that hormone replacement therapy management should aim at obtaining a thin endometrium. These data plus recent publications suggest that most women can be started on estrogen alone on a low or average dosage[32]. If the endo-

metrium thickens beyond 8 mm, a low-dose progestin should be added in a daily combination form. Sequential therapy should be the last resort, because it gives the thickest endometrium with no clear cut-off points, and gives monthly withdrawal bleeding. Sequential therapy with an endometrial thickness ~ 5 mm and no withdrawal bleeding may mean that the progestin is unnecessary.

CONCLUSIONS

Ultrasound of the endometrium is a reliable indicator of the possibility of an endometrial neoplasm. Our study, initiated because of the large supporting literature, suggests that ultrasound may be a better foundation for the management of bleeding and hormone replacement

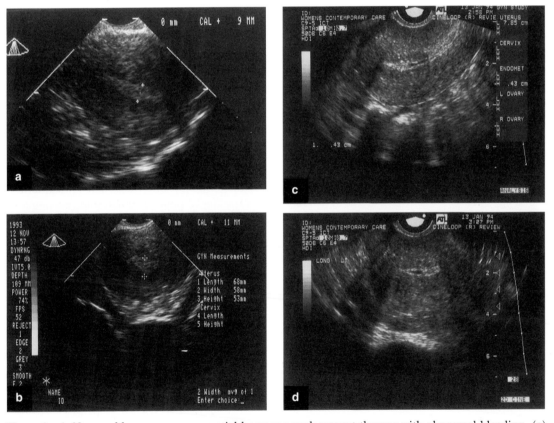

Figure 1 A 63-year-old woman on sequential hormone replacement therapy with abnormal bleeding. (a) Sagittal view of uterus showing a 9-mm endometrial lining of varying echogenicity. (b) Transverse plane showing fundal endometrium. (c) and (d) Nine weeks later without hormones, there is shrinkage of the endometrium, except for a focal thickening in the fundus. A biopsy showed a well-differentiated adenocarcinoma

therapy. Previous studies, based upon biopsy or dilatation and curettage, have sampling errors of 2–8%, and diagnostic errors up to 20% because of sampling done when the woman was still taking hormones. With ultrasound, objective management protocols can be developed for bleeding and hormone replacement therapy. Based on ultrasound studies, one goal of hormone replacement therapy should be the maintenance of a thin endometrium.

References

1. Fleischer, A. C., Kalemeris, G. C. and Machin, J. E. (1986). Sonographic depiction of normal and abnormal endometrium with histopathologic correlation. *J. Ultrasound Med.*, **5**, 445–52

2. Nasri, M. N. and Coast, G. J. (1989). Correlation of ultrasound findings and endometrial histopathology in postmenopausal women. *Br. J. Obstet. Gynaecol.*, **96**, 1333–8

3. Malpani, A., Singer, J., Wolverson, M. K. and Merenda, G. (1990). Endometrial hyperplasia: value of endometrial thickness in ultrasonographic diagnosis and clinical significance. *J. Ultrasound Med.*, **18**, 173–7

4. Schoenfeld, A., Levavi, H., Hirsch, M., Pardo, J. and Ovadia, J. (1990). Transvaginal sonography in postmenopausal women. *J. Ultrasound Med.*, **18**, 350–8

5. Osmers, R., Volksen, M., Rath, W. and Kuhn, W. (1990). Vaginosonographic detection of endometrial cancer in postmenopausal women. *Int. J. Gynecol. Obstet.*, **32**, 35–7

6. Goldstein, S. R., Nachtigall, M., Snyder, J. R. and Nachtigall, L. (1990). Endometrial assessment by vaginal ultrasonography before endometrial sampling in patients with postmenopausal bleeding. *Am. J. Obstet. Gynecol.*, **163**, 119–23

7. Rudelstorfer, R., Nanz, S. and Bernaschek, G. (1990). Vaginosonography and its diagnostic value in patients with postmenopausal bleeding. *Arch. Gynecol. Obstet.*, **248**, 37–44

8. Nasri, M. N., Shepherd, J. H., Setchell, M. E., Lowe, D. G. and Chard, T. (1991). The role of vaginal scan in measurement of endometrial thickness in postmenopausal women. *Br. J. Obstet. Gynaecol.*, **98**, 470–5

9. Smith, P., Bakos, O., Heimer, G. and Ulmsten, U. (1991). Transvaginal ultrasound for identifying endometrial abnormality. *Acta Obstet. Gynecol. Scand.*, **70**, 591–4

10. Lin, M. C., Gosink, B. B., Wolf, S. I., Feldesman, M. R., Stuenkel, C. A., Braly, P. S. and Pretorius, D. H. (1991). Endometrial thickness after menopause: effect of hormone replacement. *Radiology*, **180**, 427–32

11. Degenhardt, F., Bohmer, S., Frisch, K. and Schneider, J. (1991). Assessment of endometrium in postmenopausal women via vaginal sonography. *Ultraschall. Med.*, **12**, 119–23

12. Osmers, R., Volksen, M. and Kuhn, W. (1992). Evaluation of the endometrium in postmenopausal women by means of vaginal ultrasound. *Rev. Fr. Gynecol. Obstet.*, **87**, 309–15

13. Wikland, M., Granberg, S., and Karlsson, B. (1992). Assessment of the endometrium in the postmenopausal woman by vaginal sonography. *Ultrasound Q.*, **10**, 15–27

14. Sheth, S., Hamper, U. M. and Kurman, R. J. (1993). Thickened endometrium in the postmenopausal woman: sonographic–pathologic correlation. *Radiology*, **187**, 135–9

15. Dorum, A., Kristensen, G. B., Langebrekke, A., Sornes, T. and Skaar, O. (1993). Evaluation of endometrial thickness measured by endovaginal ultrasound in women with postmenopausal bleeding. *Acta Obstet. Gynecol. Scand.*, **72**, 116–19

16. Karlsson, B., Granberg, S., Wikland, M., Ryd, W. and Norstrom, A. (1993). Endovaginal scanning of the endometrium compared to cytology and histology in women with postmenopausal bleeding. *Gynecol. Oncol.*, **50**, 173–8

17. Wikland, M., Granberg, S. and Karlsson, B. (1993). Replacing diagnostic curettage by vaginal ultrasound. *Eur. J. Obstet. Gynecol. Reprod. Biol.*, **49**, 35–8

18. Hulka, C. A., Hall, D. A., McCarthy, K. and Simeone, J. F. (1994). Endometrial polyps, hyperplasia, and carcinoma in postmenopausal women: differentiation with endovaginal sonography. *Radiology*, **191**, 755–8

19. Shipley, C. F., III, Simmons, C. L. and Nelson, G. H. (1994). Comparison of transvaginal sonography with endometrial biopsy in asymptomatic postmenopausal women. *J. Ultrasound Med.*, **13**, 99–104

20. Holbert, T. R. (1994). Screening transvaginal ultrasonography of postmenopausal women in a private office setting. *Am. J. Obstet. Gynecol.*, **170**, 1699–704

21. Tongsong, T., Pongnarisorn, C. and Mahanuphap, P. (1994). Use of vaginosonographic measurements of endometrial thickness in the identification of abnormal endometrium in peri- and

postmenopausal bleeding. *J. Ultrasound Med.*, **22**, 479–82

22. Karlsson, B., Granberg, S., Hellberg, P., and Wikland, M. (1994). Comparative study of transvaginal sonography and hysteroscopy for the detection of pathologic endometrial lesions in women with postmenopausal bleeding. *J. Ultrasound Med.*, **13**, 757–62

23. Scarpellini, F., Curto, C., Caracussi, U., Letta, C. and Scarpellini, L. (1994). Transvaginal ultrasound versus histology in endometrial hyperplasia. *Clin. Exp. Obstet. Gynecol.*, **21**, 266–9

24. Van den Bosch, T., Vandendael, A., Van Schoubroeck, D., Wranz, P. A. B. and Lombard, C. J. (1995). Combining vaginal ultrasonography and office endometrial sampling in the diagnosis of endometrial disease in postmenopausal women. *Obstet. Gynecol.*, **85**, 349–52

25. Taipale, P., Tarjanne, H. and Heinonen, U. M. (1994). The diagnostic value of transvaginal sonography in the diagnosis of endometrial malignancy in women with peri- and postmenopausal bleeding. *Acta Obstet. Gynecol. Scand.*, **73**, 819–23

26. Kurman, R. J., Kaminski, P. F. and Norris, H. J. (1985). The behaviour of endometrial hyperplasia. A long term study of untreated hyperplasia in 170 patients. *Cancer*, **56**, 403–12

27. Baak, J. P. A., Nauta, J. J. P., Wisse-Brekelmans, E. C. M. and Bezemer, P. D. (1988). Architectural and nuclear morphometric hyperplasia features together are more important prognosticators in endometrial than nuclear morphometric features alone. *J. Pathol.*, **154**, 335–41

28. Punnonen, R., Mattila, J., Kuoppala, T. and Koivula, T. (1993). DNA ploidy, cell proliferation and steroid hormone receptors in endometrial hyperplasia and early adenocarcinoma. *J. Cancer. Res. Clin. Oncol.*, **119**, 426–9

29. Osmers, R. G., Osmers, M. and Kuhn, W. (1995). Prognostic value of transvaginal sonography in asymptomatic endometrial cancers. *Ultrasound Obstet. Gynecol.*, **6**, 103–7

30. Kurjak, A., Shalan, H., Kupesic, S., Kosuta, D., Sosic, A., Benic, S., Ilijas, M., Jukic, S. and Predanic, M. (1994). An attempt to screen asymptomatic women for ovarian and endometrial cancer with transvaginal color and pulsed Doppler sonography. *J. Ultrasound Med.*, **13**, 295–301

31. Schulman, H., Conway, C., Zalud, I., Farmakides, G., Haley, J. and Cassata, M. (1994). Prevalence in a volunteer population of pelvic cancer detected with transvaginal ultrasound and color flow Doppler. *Ultrasound Obstet. Gynecol.*, **4**, 414–20

32. Dubinsky, T. J., Parvey, R., Gormaz, G., Curtis, M. and Maklad, N. J. (1995). Transvaginal hysterosonography: comparison with biopsy in the evaluation of postmenopausal bleeding. *Ultrasound Med.*, **14**, 887–93

33. ACOG Committee Opinion. Number 126, August 1993. Estrogen replacement therapy and endometrial cancer

34. ACOG Committee Opinion. Number 169, February 1996. Tamoxifen and endometrial cancer

35. Grady, D., Gebretsadik, T., Kerlikowske, K., Ernster, V. and Petitti, D. (1995). Hormone replacement therapy and endometrial cancer risk: a meta-analysis. *Obstet. Gynecol.*, **85**, 304–13

36. Udoff, L., Langenberg, P. and Adashi, E. Y. (1995). Combined continuous hormone replacement therapy: a critical review. *Obstet. Gynecol.*, **86**, 306–16

37. Spicer, K. V. and Pike, M. (1995). Hormonal manipulation to prevent breast cancer. *Sci. Am. Sci. Med.*, **2**, 58–67

38. Woodruff, J. D., Pickar, J. H., for the Menopause Study Group. (1994). Incidence of endometrial hyperplasia in postmenopausal women taking conjugated estrogens (Premarin) with medroxyprogesterone or conjugated estrogens alone. *Am. J. Obstet. Gynecol.*, **170**, 1213–23

39. Writing Group for the PEPI Trial (1996). Effects of hormone replacement therpay on endometrial histology in postmenopausal women. The postmenopausal estrogen/progestin interventions (PEPI) Trial. *J. Am. Med. Assoc.*, **275**, 370–5

40. Zalud, I., Conway, C., Schulman, H. and Tinca, D. (1993). Endometrial and myometrial thickness and uterine blood flow in postmenopausal women: the influence of hormonal replacement therapy and age. *J. Ultrasound Med.*, **12**, 7341

41. Bonilla-Musoles, F., Ballester, M. J., Marti, M. C., Raga, F. and Osborne, N. G. (1995). Transvaginal color Doppler assessment of endometrial status in normal postmenopausal women: the effect of hormone replacement therapy. *J. Ultrasound Med.*, **14**, 491–6

42. Ferenczy, A. and Gelfand, M. (1989). The biologic significance of cytologic atypia in progestogen treated endometrial hyperplasia. *Am. J. Obstet. Gynecol.*, **160**, 126–31

43. Ettinger, B. (1993). Use of low dosage 17 beta estradiol for the prevention of osteoporosis. *Clin. Ther.*, **15**, 950–62

44. Ismail, A. A. A., Ramadan, M., Soliman, A., Rahmy, A. and Rizk, A. (1988). Postmenopausal endometrial patterns and serum estradiol concentrations. *Int. J. Gynaecol. Obstet.*, **27**, 101–5

45. Sauer, M. V., Miles, R. A., Dahmoush, L., Paulson, R. J., Press, M. and Moyer, D. (1993). Evaluating the effect of age on endometrial responsiveness to hormone replacement therapy: a histologic ultrasonographic, and tissue receptor analysis. *J. Assist. Reprod. Genet.*, **10**, 47–52

Transvaginal sonography of endometrial disorders in postmenopausal women

4

S. Granberg, T. H. Bourne, M. Wikland, M. Hahlin, B. Gull and B. Karlsson

INTRODUCTION

With the development and clinical application of transvaginal transducers/probes, the sonographic imaging of the endometrium was greatly enhanced compared with abdominal ultrasound. Also, the discomfort of a full bladder associated with abdominal ultrasound could be avoided. A shorter distance between probe and target allowed the use of higher-frequency transducers, thereby achieving improved imaging.

Wild and Reid constructed a transvaginal rigid transducer in the mid 1950s[1]. Based on the work by Wild and Reid, the use of transvaginal sonography (TVS) was first reported by Kratochwil in 1969[2]. However, due to technical problems, the development of TVS was delayed and the use of high-frequency transvaginal transducers for clinical routine use was first reported by Schwimmer and Lebovic in 1984[3].

This chapter will only discuss the use of TVS, but this does not mean that abdominal ultrasound should not or cannot be used when dealing with the postmenopausal uterus.

Transvaginal sonography provides a valuable tool for the diagnosis of a wide range of gynecological disorders including those of the uterus and endometrium. The ability of TVS to depict the thickness and morphology of the endometrium has been established in both office and hospital settings. This article will discuss and illustrate the clinical and research applications of TVS in relation to the endometrium in both symptomatic and asymptomatic postmenopausal women. The article is of particular relevance today given the number of women who are undergoing transvaginal ultrasono-graphy in the absence of symptoms as a part of their routine check-ups. There is a paucity of data relating to the management of apparent ultrasound abnormalities in such women.

In symptomatic women, or for women at risk of developing endometrial pathology, a technique that could reduce the number of biopsy procedures would be of value. Hysteroscopy, dilatation and curettage (D&C) as well as other endometrial sampling methods are all invasive; thus it would be of benefit if a way could be found to assess the endometrium using a relatively non-invasive approach. Such a technique would need to be relatively easy to learn and perform, as well as being well accepted by the patients. We believe that transvaginal sonography fulfils many of these requirements; the following review will attempt to put forward some of the evidence to support this view.

METHODOLOGY AND TVS MEASUREMENT OF THE ENDOMETRIUM

It is important to define precisely what we mean when we talk about endometrial thickness. For the purposes of this review, it is the maximal total measurement that can be obtained across the lumen of the cavity from one endometrial–myometrial interface to another. This measurement excludes intracavity fluid, but includes any tissue (Figure 1). This measurement will usually be taken just below the fundus. Hence, endometrial thickness actually relates to two 'endometria'. If the use of certain cut-off values

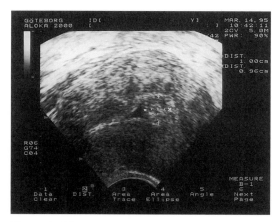

Figure 1 Measurement of the endometrial cavity including a polyp (10 mm) in a retroverted uterus. Orientation, longitudinal scan; transducer's tip at the bottom of the figure

derived from the measurement of endometrial thickness using TVS is ever to be widely accepted as a method for excluding endometrial pathology in women with postmenopausal bleeding, then the issue of reproducibility will be of vital importance. This may be particularly relevant with respect to operators with different levels of experience with ultrasound.

In order to address this question, we performed a study whereby the interobserver variation between one experienced and five inexperienced TVS examiners was evaluated[4]. After pooling the data from all the inexperienced examiners, there was a good correlation between the measurements obtained by the experienced and the inexperienced operators. A total of 90 pairs of measurements were obtained from 90 women and the mean difference between the two measurements on each woman was 1.5 mm. In 51% of the data-pairs, the experienced and inexperienced doctors recorded the same measurements. However, if the measurements from each inexperienced examiner were considered individually and compared with those from the experienced user, there was a considerable difference between the measurements obtained. Two of the five inexperienced examiners were able to measure the endometrial thickness very accurately whilst the other three produced measurements at considerable variance with the 'true' endometrial

thickness. This is perhaps not surprising since it is known that some people have a natural affinity towards the interpretation of ultrasound images, whilst others need more training. This illustrates the importance of a certain period of supervision for those who are to perform endometrial measurements using TVS. The tendency to ignore supervision and training in gynecological ultrasound is to be deprecated given the potentially serious consequences of an incorrect interpretation of a scan on patient management. In a study by Cohen and co-workers, it was suggested that the variation of the measurements of the endometrium obtained most often was due to different assessment of the endometrial–myometrial junction, selection of different imaging views, or actual variation in the endometrial thickness due to uterine contractility[5].

Karlsson and co-workers concluded that measurements of the endometrial thickness by TVS in women with postmenopausal bleeding can be performed reproducibly after a certain period of training. However, the period of training will vary from operator to operator[4]. It seems reasonable to conclude that, during the first 25–50 measurements of the endometrial thickness by TVS, an experienced examiner should be available for supervision. It was also quite clear that, in women with submucous myomas, it was more difficult to measure the endometrial thickness[4]. Furthermore, as with other reports, we found that it is difficult to make an assessment of the degree of myometrial invasion of a particular carcinoma[6–8].

The fact that neither an experienced nor an inexperienced examiner will always be able to identify the endometrium by TVS makes it important to consider such a TVS finding to be potentially pathological. If it is not possible to identify the endometrial cavity clearly, then hydrosonography should be performed (see later in text for details). If the endometrium still cannot be visualized, then an invasive biopsy procedure is indicated in order to rule out pathology. That an invasive cancer may make it difficult to image the cavity gives emphasis to this point. The fact that it is not always possible to identify the endometrium by TVS is illustrated by the study by Auslender and colleagues who reported an endometrial thickness (double layer) in the range of 0–6.5 mm for women with postmenopausal bleeding[9]. The zero must represent an endometrium that could not be measured. A measurement of zero is also used in a study by Bakos and colleagues, where an endometrial thickness of 0 mm was obtained in women with apparent atrophic endometrium, where no tissue was obtained or in endometria that was hormonally affected according to the histopathological diagnosis at D&C[10].

When using ultrasound, it is of great importance to be certain that what is believed to represent the endometrium is in fact just that. In a study by Nasri and Coast, the endometrial thickness was measured in ten women using TVS prior to hysterectomy for cervical intraepithelial neoplasia (CIN). The ultrasound measurements were within 1.0 mm of the actual thickness taken from the fresh unfixed specimen[11]. Karlsson and co-workers, in a series of 25 women, also compared TVS measurements of endometrial thickness before hysterectomy with pathological findings. They found that the mean difference between the measurement obtained by ultrasound and that from the pathologist's ruler was 3.3 mm[4]. The most probable explanation for the thinner endometrial measurements obtained from hysterectomy specimens is that the uterus actually shrinks when it is not perfused. However, it is reassuring that, if anything, transvaginal ultrasound tends to overestimate the real endometrial thickness. Hence, it is unlikely that any major pathology will be missed.

STANDARD TECHNIQUES FOR ASSESSING THE ENDOMETRIUM AS COMPARED TO TRANSVAGINAL ULTRASOUND

Bleeding from the genital tract after the menopause has and is always regarded as an indication to perform some kind of endometrial biopsy. For many years the most widely used technique for obtaining a sample of endometrium for histological evaluation has been by D&C. However, this test has well-recognized limitations. Several studies have questioned the sensitivity and specificity of curettage for the detection of endometrial disease in comparison to other endometrial biopsy techniques that are available[12–19]. It has previously been reported that D&C has a false-negative rate of between 2% and 6% for diagnosing endometrial cancer and hyperplasia[12–19]. Such figures hold true for less invasive 'outpatient' methods of obtaining an endometrial sample such as the Vabra (Berkeley Medevices, Berkeley, CA, USA) and Pipelle (Milex Products, Chicago, IL, USA)[13,17,20]. Perhaps the main reason for these problems is that of sampling error. As it is a 'blind' procedure, in approximately 60% of D&Cs, less than half of the uterine cavity is actually curetted[19]. Stock and Kanbour demonstrated this point by performing a D&C immediately prior to hysterectomy in 50 women[19]. They showed that, in 30 out of the 50 patients (60%), less than half of the cavity was sampled[19]. In a further study, Stovall and co-workers found that D&C before hysterectomy missed 5.7% of cases of hyperplasia and endometrial cancer[21]. The same authors reported that endometrial pathology was missed in 4% when the Novak biopsy technique was used[21]. We have had similar experience. In a study of 185 women, we found that D&C was associated with a false-negative rate of 2.2% when the histological sample taken at D&C was compared to subsequent hysterectomy specimens[22]. It is clear, therefore, that the use of the D&C as a 'gold standard' for the assessment of endometrial pathology has serious limitations.

More recently, the evaluation of endometrial pathology under direct vision has become possible with the advent of hysteroscopes that can be used in the office environment. This also offers the advantage of enabling the operator to take directed biopsies. The theoretical risk of sampling errors should therefore be reduced. However, this presupposes that the operator will recognize areas of endometrial abnormality under direct vision when they are there. This is not always the case. Furthermore, many outpatient hysteroscopes have no operating channel with which to take biopsies, and so sampling is still in effect 'blind'. However, the literature suggests that in many cases hysteroscopy will provide an increase in diagnostic information. Gimpleson and Rappold[23] studied 276 patients who underwent both hysteroscopy and D&C. Hysteroscopy yielded more information in 44 patients whilst D&C gave more accurate information in only nine patients. The use of hysteroscopy seemed to offer particular advantages with respect to the diagnosis of endometrial polyps and submucous myomas. Several patients in this study underwent multiple curettage procedures before their endometrial pathology was revealed using the hysteroscope[23]. These data are further supported by a study by Townsend and co-workers who found, using hysteroscopy, that almost 90% of women with persistent postmenopausal bleeding had either polyps or submucous myomas as the primary cause of their bleeding[24]. It would therefore seem that it is against hysteroscopy that TVS must be compared if its true role in the assessment of the postmenopausal uterus is to be found.

ASSESSMENT OF UTERUS IN THE PRESENCE OF POSTMENOPAUSAL BLEEDING BY TRANSVAGINAL ULTRASOUND

When addressing this issue, it is important that the full potential of TVS in this context is realized. Virtually all the data relating to this clinical situation refer to the use of TVS without the use of negative contrast media. More recently, the introduction of hydrosonography has probably led to a significant increase in the diagnostic accuracy of TVS in this context[25–27]. Where the precise character of the endometrial echo obtained during a scan is unclear, the instillation of a negative contrast medium in the form of sterile saline into the cavity will often give excellent views of the cavity and allow a diagnosis to be made. The saline is infused through a fine flexible catheter into the cavity whilst the transvaginal scan is performed. Thus the presence or absence of polyps or cavity irregularities can be seen clearly in 'real time' (Figure 2). The saline acts both to distend the cavity and to provide an acoustic window to the walls of the endometrial cavity. This technique seems to hold particular

promise in the diagnosis of polyps and submucous myomas. Bourne and colleagues have described the use of this technique as a novel approach to the diagnosis of polyps associated with tamoxifen therapy[27]. Sterile saline is slowly infused into the uterine cavity under direct ultrasound control. This technique will reveal both polyps and irregularities of the endometrial cavity and could thus be an alternative to hysteroscopy[27]. The situation discussed earlier when it is difficult to delineate the endometrial cavity is a further indication for the use of this technique.

It can be estimated that about 10% of women with postmenopausal bleeding will subsequently be found to harbor an endometrial carcinoma[14,16,21]. Furthermore, of the remainder, about 20–40% will have either hyperplasia, an endometrial polyp, or some other form of endometrial pathology as the cause of their bleeding. Therefore the majority of women with postmenopausal bleeding (50–60%) will be bleeding because of a benign condition, that will be confirmed as such on biopsy. Once a cervical lesion has been excluded, the cause of these women's bleeding is usually considered to be fragile blood vessels in the thin atrophic mucosa of the endometrium and/or vaginal skin[28]. The argument in favor of developing an ultrasound-based test that could effectively rule out serious

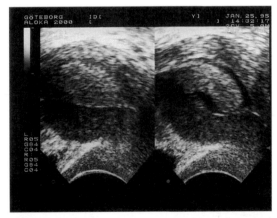

Figure 2 Left image shows a thick endometrium. Right image shows a polyp visualized at hydrosonography and a thin atrophic endometrium. Orientation, longitudinal scan; transducer's tip at the bottom of the figure

pathology in the majority of women with post-menopausal bleeding, thus saving them an invasive biopsy procedure, has engendered considerable interest.

IS THERE ANY CUT-OFF VALUE FOR DETECTING ENDOMETRIAL PATHOLOGY BY TRANSVAGINAL ULTRASOUND?

In order to define the presence or absence of pathology, it is necessary to make the test less subjective and generate some quantitative data. We must therefore address the issue of whether endometrial thickness cut-off values exist that can be used to ascertain the likelihood of pathology being present in the endometrial cavity. In particular, it is of interest to know the negative predictive value of a thin endometrium measured using ultrasound.

In a study of postmenopausal women without uterine bleeding, we found a mean endometrial thickness of 3.2 mm[29]. This figure is in agreement with other reports in the literature on similar groups of women[28-36]. We subsequently reported that the mean endometrial thickness for women with postmenopausal bleeding but with a histopathological diagnosis of atrophy was 3.4 mm[34] (Figure 3). However, in the Nordic endometrial trial of over 1000 women with postmenopausal bleeding, the corresponding figure

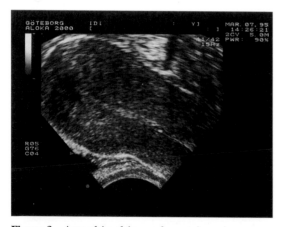

Figure 3 Atrophic thin endometrium in an anteverted uterus. Women with postmenopausal bleeding. Orientation, longitudinal scan; transducer's tip at the bottom of the figure

was found to be 3.9 mm (range 1–22 mm)[33]. These results are consistent with other studies relating to symptomatic postmenopausal women[9,10,28-30]. The data relating to endometrial thickness in the presence of carcinoma also demonstrate a marked degree of concordance. Of particular interest is the fact that few if any carcinomas have been observed with an endometrial thickness of less than 5.0 mm[9,32].

A selective view of the literature can allow one to quote 11 published studies involving almost 2500 women with postmenopausal bleeding examined by TVS. No endometrial cancer has been found in a uterus whose endometrium measured below 5.0 mm[28-31,33-40]. However, there have been exceptions that deserve attention. There have been two studies where endometrial cancer has been reported in women with an endometrial thickness of less than 5 mm as measured by TVS[32,41]. Abu-Hmeidan and colleagues described five such cancers amongst 571 women with postmenopausal bleeding[41], whilst Dörum and co-workers included two amongst their series of 100 symptomatic women[32]. However, some of these data are somewhat inconsistent. For example, in the study by Dörum and colleagues, one stage Ic cancer was reported with an endometrial thickness of only 3.0 mm[32]. Given the staging criteria for endometrial cancer, stage Ic implies that more than 50% of the myometrium has been infiltrated by cancer. An endometrial thickness measurement of just 3.0 mm is not credible under these circumstances, and must represent a measurement error using ultrasound. However, operator error is an integral part of any ultrasound examination and cannot be excluded from any analysis of overall test performance. This case highlights the difficulties that can be encountered when identifying the myometrial–endometrial interface in the presence of invasive disease. It must be emphasized that, if the endometrium cannot be clearly delineated even after hydrosonography, then this is an indication for invasive biopsy. It also stresses the need for thorough training in the method of measuring the endometrial thickness by means of TVS. As with any cut-off values used in differentiating the normal from the abnormal, it is inevitable that false-negative test results will occur when a value of 5.0 mm is used. However, according to the multicenter Nordic study, which includes over 1160 women, as well as the data referred to above, the risk of malignancy within ultrasonically measured thin endometrium is low.

Another important point alluded to above that came out of the Nordic study was that, rather like the postmenopausal ovary, a failure to visualize the structure under investigation does not imply normality. In obstetric practice, this is rather like saying that if you cannot get a view of the heart it probably does not matter. Yet failure to see pelvic structures in gynecology is not uncommon. This rather *laissez-faire* attitude to gynecological ultrasound probably reflects the fact that many of the people involved in ultrasound in obstetrics and gynecology come from an obstetric ultrasound background, and in fact have a limited regard and knowledge of the applications of ultrasound in gynecology. In the Nordic trial, 2.8% (*n* = 33) of the women had an endometrium which could not be measured[30]. Subsequent histology of endometrial biopsies revealed that nine of these women had endometrial pathology, including one endometrial cancer. Ignoring endometrium that cannot be visualized on ultrasound is not acceptable practice. Although the use of an endometrial thickness cut-off value of < 5.0 mm seems reasonable to select those women at low risk of harboring a malignancy, it is also important to consider other pathology. Again we can consider data from the Nordic trial. Fourteen women with an endometrium measuring < 5 mm (2.7% of all women with an endometrial thickness < 5 mm) were found to have endometrial pathology other than cancer[33]. This figure may be compared with the false-negative results obtained with D&C, reported to be up to 10%[12,14,18-21]. These data are in agreement with other reports where polyps and hyperplasia have been found in endometria measuring 5 mm or less[28,40,42]. The percentage of polyps (Figure 4) or hyperplasia (Figure 5) found in these small series after D&C in the group of women with an endometrial thickness < 5 mm varies between 0 and 14%[28,40,42]. Whether hydrosonography might be used to improve the overall test

performance has yet to be determined; however, it is quite conceivable that it might lead to an improvement in the detection of endometrial polyps in this particular cohort of women[25-27]. The results from the Nordic study have recently been reproduced by an Italian multicenter trial, by Ferrazzi and colleagues[43].

So is the use of a cut-off value of less than 5.0 mm reasonable? Certainly our data[30] as well as the data presented by Ferrazzi and colleagues[43] support its use in women with postmenopausal bleeding. A statistical analysis to calculate the probability of there being endometrial pathology present at a certain

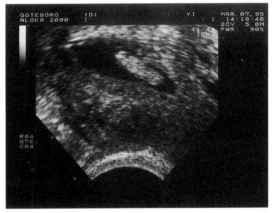

Figure 4 Small polyp visualized in a woman with postmenopausal bleeding and a thin endometrium (4 mm). Orientation, longitudinal scan; transducer's tip at the bottom of the figure

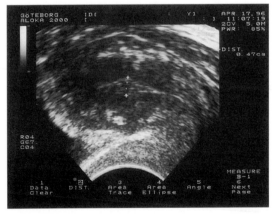

Figure 5 Hyperplasia without atypia in a woman with postmenopausal bleeding (5 mm). Orientation, transducer's tip at the bottom of the figure

endometrial thickness value shows that the risk of overlooking an endometrial abnormality at an endometrial thickness of < 5.0 mm is 5.5%. The corresponding figure for < 6 mm is 8.5%. The receiver–operator curve and a calculation of the probability that a pathological diagnosis will be overlooked at certain levels of endometrial thickness indicate that the cut-off limit < 5.0 mm is suitable for excluding an endometrial abnormality. The calculated risk of 5.5% (upper confidence limit) of missing pathology at this limit compares favorably with the false-negative rate quoted for D&C of 4–6%[14,16–21]. However, by selecting women with postmenopausal bleeding for further investigation on the basis of an endometrial thickness of 5.0 mm or more, we would be able to reduce the number of biopsy procedures by 46% (see Tables 1 and 2).

ENDOMETRIAL CAVITY FLUID

A further consideration in any morphological assessment of the endometrium is the presence or absence of intracavity fluid. It has been claimed that endometrial cavity fluid (Figure 6) is associated with an increased risk of endometrial and other pelvic pathology[44]. The conclusion of this paper was that all postmenopausal women with endometrial cavity fluid should undergo an endometrial biopsy procedure. In contrast, our experience has not mirrored the findings of this study (Figure 7). In a follow-up study of 50 asymptomatic postmenopausal women found to have fluid within the endometrial cavity, no malignant disease was found at the time of hysteroscopy after a follow-up period of 1 year[45]. Our anecdotal experience has also been that it is not unusual for cavity fluid to be present within the endometrial cavity of women taking hormone replacement therapy, particularly in the progestogen phase of cyclical therapy. It is not our policy to perform endometrial biopsies on women with intracavity fluid in the absence of symptoms.

Table 1 Endometrial thickness related to the histopathological diagnosis of atrophy in women with postmenopausal bleeding, in some published papers

Reference	Thickness (mean ± SD) (mm)	Range (mm)
Granberg et al. (1988)[29]*	3.2 ± 1.1	1–8
Granberg et al. (1991)[34]	3.4 ± 1.2	2–11
Bourne et al. (1991)[48]	8.0 ± 1.1	2–16
Bourne et al. (1991)[48]*	4.0 ± 2.0	2–15
Botsis et al. (1992)[31]	3.2 ± 1.1	—
Auslender et al. (1993)[9]	2.6 ± 1.4	0–6.5
Dörum et al. (1993)[32]	4.0	1–9
Bakos et al. (1994)[10]	4.6	0–10
Karlsson et al.(1994)[4]	3.9 ± 2.5	1–22

*Asymptomatic postmenopausal women without postmenopausal bleeding
Table from the thesis of T. Bourne, 1995

Table 2 Endometrial thickness related to the histopathological diagnosis of endometrial carcinoma in women with postmenopausal bleeding, in some published papers

Reference	Thickness (mean ± SD) (mm)	Range (mm)
Granberg et al. (1991)[34]	18.2 ± 6.2	9–35
Bourne et al. (1991)[48]	20.0 ± 9.0	6–41
Botsis et al. (1992)[31]	16.6 ± 5.4	—
Auslender et al. (1993)[9]	18.1 ± 9.2	7–40
Dörum et al. (1993)[32]	20	2–30
Bakos et al. (1994)[10]	13.9	6–31
Karlsson et al. (1994)[4]	21.1 ± 11.8	5–68

Table from the thesis of T. Bourne, 1995

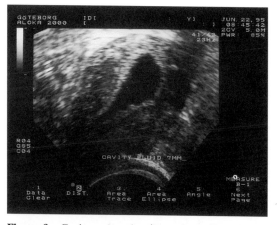

Figure 6 Cavity measuring 7 mm including the cavity fluid. The thickness of the endometrium was 1 mm on both sides. Orientation, transducer's tip at the bottom of the figure

TRANSVAGINAL COLOR DOPPLER IN THE CONTEXT OF ENDOMETRIAL PATHOLOGY

It should already be clear from this article that B-mode imaging will provide a wealth of useful information about the postmenopausal endometrium.

However, whilst there are now good data to suggest that the measurements of endometrial thickness made using transvaginal ultrasonography can have a high negative predictive value for malignancy, there is a significant false-

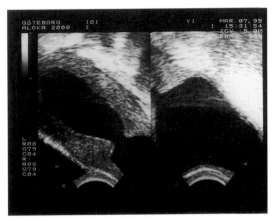

Figure 7 Hematometra and 'cervixometra'. Note the internal os of the cervix. The histopathological diagnosis was atrophy and hematometra. There was a cervical stenosis due to a Manchester operation, including amputation of cervix uteri. Orientation, longitudinal scan; transducer's tip at the bottom of the figure

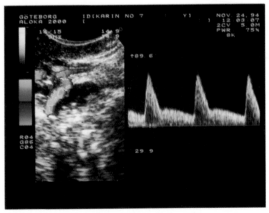

Figure 8 Uterine arteries. Orientation, transducer's tip at the bottom of the figure

positive rate. It has been suggested that an assessment of uterine vascularity may provide information that could improve overall test performance.

The characteristic flow velocity waveforms that can be obtained from the uterine artery have been described (Figure 8). Recent reports have suggested that transvaginal color Doppler can be used to measure reproducibly impedance to blood flow in these vessels[46,47]. Using the pulsatility index (PI), a one-way analysis of variance of replicate data from 20 women has given coefficients of variation of the order of 10% for both uterine arteries (Figure 7).

Bourne and colleagues[48] measured impedance to blood flow in the uterine arteries as well as endometrial thickness in women with postmenopausal bleeding both with and without cancer, as well as women taking hormone replacement therapy and those thought to have a normal uterus taking no drug therapy. The information relating to endometrial thickness generated by this study is in broad agreement with those discussed above. However, one important finding was the fact that the endometrial thickness for women taking hormone replacement therapy was increased relative to those not on therapy. Hence, cut-off values derived from the populations of asymptomatic women already discussed in this review are unlikely to apply. Data from this study suggest that, in the presence of malignant tissue, the impedance to uterine artery blood flow is reduced significantly when compared to control groups. In all cases of endometrial carcinoma, the uterine artery PI measured less than 1.8. Impedance to blood flow in the uterine arteries increases with years from the menopause, and so these results cannot be explained by differences in patient age. It may be that this difference can be accounted for by the presence of neovascularization in the endometrial cavity, or possibly because these women are inherently more sensitive to the action of endogenous estrogens. This may predispose them to the development of endometrial carcinoma as well as being associated with a decreased impedance to flow in the uterine arteries secondary to vasodilatation. Using color Doppler, the false-positive rate of the B-mode ultrasound-based test was reduced whilst maintaining sensitivity. Perhaps of more clinical value is that, if color Doppler is used to interrogate the endometrium in the presence of carcinoma, angiogenesis can be demonstrated as areas of color superimposed on the B-mode gray-scale image and the sensitivity of the technique may be enhanced. The area where color Doppler may have most value would be in examining the uterus in cases where the endometrium is thickened to search for areas of angiogenesis (Figure 9). An interesting further observation in this study was that there was a marked reduction in blood flow impedance within the uterine arteries of women taking hormone replacement therapy, a point that will be discussed later in this article.

Other workers have also reported vascular changes in the presence of uterine cancer using color Doppler. In one report, two cases of endometrial cancer were examined, and resistance index (RI) values from the periphery of the endometrial echo were 0.26 and 0.31, respectively[49]. Hata and co-workers[50] examined ten women with endometrial cancer and found areas of low impedance blood flow in all cases (PI 0.535 ± 0.158); in patients with uterine myomata the intratumoral blood flow impedance was 0.679 ± 0.131. Attempts have been made to characterize uterine tumors using transvaginal color Doppler[51]. Intratumoral blood flow was looked for in 291 benign and 17 malignant uterine tumors. The RI value was 0.58 ± 0.12 SD for cases of uterine myomata, and 0.34 ± 0.03 in cases of endometrial carcinoma. The authors conclude that transvaginal color Doppler can be used to help discriminate between benign and malignant uterine tumors, and that an intratumoral RI value of < 0.40 should be regarded as malignant and between 0.40 and 0.50 as suspicious. In general, the ultrasound appearances of myomata and endometrial carcinoma are distinct and quite different, and to what extent color Doppler will ever be necessary to discriminate between the two is uncertain. Our experience with fibroids suggests that low-impedance high-velocity blood flow is a normal finding from such tumors[52] and outside the context of research we do not believe that color Doppler has a useful role in this area. The observation in the same report that a uterine sarcoma (RI 0.31) had significantly lower impedance blood flow than benign myomata may, if substantiated, have more practical clinical implications. However, our anecdotal findings have been that such low-impedance flow in fibroids is not uncommon, and we do not believe that this is likely to indicate the presence of a sarcoma.

More recently, Weiner and colleagues reported significantly lower RI values from the uterine arteries of women with endometrial pathology than in women with no pathological findings of the endometrium[42]. In a further study Bourne and co-workers[53] used transvaginal color Doppler to assess uterine blood flow and morphology in 227 postmenopausal women. Seventy-two had symptoms of postmenopausal bleeding and 155 were asymptomatic. All these women underwent endometrial biopsy after the Doppler scan. In this study, all women with endometrial cancer had a significantly thicker endometrium (mean 20.2 mm) than the other groups, such as those with atrophic endometrium (mean 1.35 mm). In addition, all cases of uterine cancer had a markedly lower pulsatility index (PI 1.00 compared to 3.80 for atrophic endometrium). Once again, we found that women taking hormone replacement therapy demonstrated a marked

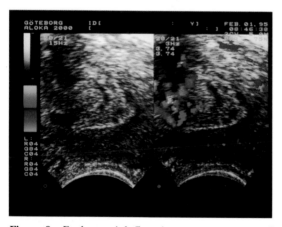

Figure 9 Endometrial flow in a postmenopausal endometrium. Histopathological diagnosis was hyperplasia without atypia. Orientation, transducer's tip at the bottom of the figure

decrease in impedance to blood flow in the uterine arteries (mean 2.5), suggesting that estrogens may have a direct effect on the human vasculature.

So, does color Doppler have a clinical role in the assessment of the postmenopausal uterus? Whilst the data discussed above (including our own) suggest that there might be differences in uterine artery blood flow between those with and without serious endometrial pathology, in practical terms we do not believe color Doppler has a significant role to play. The reality is that the finding of thickened endometrium in a symptomatic woman will lead to an endometrial biopsy irrespective of the color Doppler findings. Furthermore, no large-scale studies have been performed to evaluate the benefits of color flow imaging over TVS with measurement of the endometrial thickness as the sole parameter indicating endometrial abnormality. For the present time, although its research potential is unquestioned, color Doppler findings should not be used to influence clinical practice. For those practitioners who do not have access to a color Doppler machine for their gynecological ultrasound examinations, we would not advise that you try too hard to find one – it is unlikely to change your management of patients.

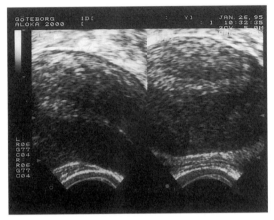

Figure 10 Women on HRT with a benign endometrium. To the left longitudinal scan and to the right transverse scan. Orientation, transducer's tip at the bottom of the figure

HORMONAL EFFECTS ON THE POSTMENOPAUSAL ENDOMETRIUM

Hormone replacement therapy

B-mode imaging

Changes in both the thickness and texture of the fertile endometrium have been observed during follicular maturation in both spontaneous and stimulated menstrual cycles[46]. It seems that under the influence of exogenous hormones the postmenopausal endometrium also undergoes cyclical changes which can be visualized by TVS (Figures 10–12).

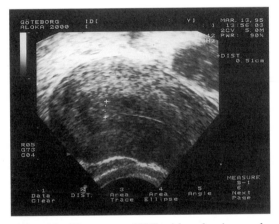

Figure 11 Women on HRT with a benign endometrium. Note the triple-line pattern. Orientation, transducer's tip at the bottom of the figure

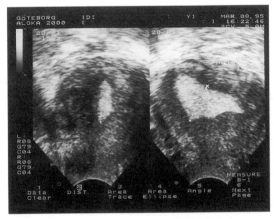

Figure 12 Women on HRT with a benign endometrium. Longitudinal and transverse scan. Note the hyperechogenic endometrium. Orientation, transducer's tip at the bottom of the figure

We followed 54 postmenopausal women from the start of hormone replacement therapy (HRT) treatment up to 1 year. An endometrial sample was taken prior to starting therapy and again 1 year later. All women received a cyclical progestogen (10 mg daily) for 12 days of each calendar month. The mean endometrial thickness prior to starting HRT was 2.8 ± 1.1 mm (range 1–5 mm). One year later during the progestogen phase of the cycle it was 4.2 ± 1.7 mm (range 1–9 mm) and 2–4 days after progestin treatment 3.1 ± 1.5 mm (range 1–5 mm). It also seemed that the use of HRT is associated with a significant increase in uterine volume after 1 year of treatment[54].

A further study has also demonstrated an increase in endometrial thickness in women taking HRT. In this study by Gull and associates[55], a random sample of postmenopausal women in Göteborg were examined using transvaginal ultrasonography. Three hundred and twenty-eight out of 364 postmenopausal women not receiving any HRT (90%) had an endometrial thickness ≤ 4 mm, 25 (7%) had a thickness of 5–7 mm and in 11 women (3%) the endometrial thickness as measured by TVS was ≥ 8 mm. The corresponding figures for those women receiving HRT were 49%, 42% and 9% and for those taking estriol they were 86%, 7% and 7%. Put simply, a greater proportion of women on HRT tend to have an increase in endometrial thickness than those who do not. However, these data do not take into account cycle day, nor the specific type of therapy given. A closer analysis of these results shows a significant variation in endometrial thickness according to which phase of cyclical therapy the patient was examined on. From 'cycle day' 1–7 the mean endometrial thickness was 4.3 mm, 'cycle day' 8–14 it was 6.8 mm, 'cycle day' 15–21 it was 6.0 mm and 'cycle day' 22–28 it was 6.2 mm. It is clear that finding 'thick' endometrium in women on HRT is a normal finding. It is probably best to examine such women immediately after their withdrawal bleed when the endometrium should be at its thinnest. It might be hypothesized that a thick endometrium that does not change following progestogen therapy might be more likely to harbor pathology; how-

ever, there are few data to substantiate this view. Women taking HRT who develop abnormal bleeding should be investigated by biopsy. The data relating to endometrial thickness for women on HRT are too scanty to manage the patient on the basis of ultrasound criteria. Nevertheless, Lin and co-workers[56] have suggested that women receiving HRT who are found to have an endometrium measuring ≥ 8 mm should undergo further investigation in the form of an endometrial biopsy. Our data tend to support this view, although we would advocate a repeat scan in the immediate postmenopausal phase of the cycle first.

Monitoring the effects of estrogen on the endometrium by TVS has recently been suggested by Meuvissen and colleagues[57]. They have postulated that the endometrial thickness as measured by TVS can be used almost as a biological assay of endometrial response to exogenous estrogens. This makes the assumption that endometrial proliferation, hyperplasia, or cancer will always be associated with an increase in endometrial thickness. In this way it might be possible to select those women who do not need as much progestogen therapy as others to counter the effects of estrogens. In the absence of a significant increase in endometrial thickness in response to estrogens, it might be possible not to give a progestogen. In the presence of significant endometrial growth (> 3 mm), progestogen should be added. By identifying women with 'fast growing' as opposed to 'slow growing' endometrium it may be possible to select those women whose endometria are sensitive to the effects of exogenous estrogen, and thus at risk of developing an endometrial abnormality. This is an attractive concept that still needs to be substantiated by further studies before being introduced into clinical practice[57].

Recently Levine and associates[58] published a paper ($n = 120$ postmenopausal women) where they concluded that women using sequential hormones show greater endometrial thickness than non-users and show the most variation in measurements. Furthermore, they concluded that these women should undergo ultrasound either early or late in the hormone cycle to evaluate the endometrium at its thinnest[58].

Blood flow and HRT

Transvaginal color Doppler has been used to show that estrogens reduce impedance to blood flow in the uterine artery by 50%[37]. If extrapolated to the general vasculature, this would have obvious implications with regard to the cardioprotective effect of estrogen replacement therapy. The changes in uterine artery impedance occurred rapidly. A protein related to the estradiol receptor has been identified in the intima of major vessels[59], and it is possible that estrogens affect arterial status through a conventional sex hormone–receptor mechanism. The addition of progestogens appears partially to reverse this drop in impedance, although not to pretreatment levels[60]; this takes effect within 36 h of starting progestogen therapy, suggesting that the mechanism is also receptor-mediated[61]. A particularly interesting observation in the study by Hillard and colleagues[60] was that the response to exogenous estrogens was proportional to the number of years since the menopause. If this is confirmed, there may be cardiovascular benefit from estrogen administration even in very elderly women, as they may still have a significant vascular response to therapy. Selecting progestogens that have the least effect on the vasodilatation brought about by estrogen therapy may be of great importance if the beneficial effects of hormone replacement therapy are to be maximized; such a choice may be investigated with the use of transvaginal color Doppler. These data were later supported by those of de Ziegler and co-workers[62]. In six women with either idiopathic premature ovarian failure or ovarian failure secondary to chemotherapy, uterine artery blood flow was assessed before and during estrogen therapy. The PI before treatment was 5.2 ± 0.4 (mean $\pm$ SEM), dropping to 1.3 ± 0.3 when taking exogenous estrogens. Studies of other vessels have now shown similar changes in response to estrogen therapy[63]. Doppler ultrasonography of the aorta has demonstrated that estrogens increase both stroke volume and flow acceleration. These are thought to reflect a combination of inotropism and vasodilatation. Changes in uterine artery response to exogenous estrogens seem to act as a model for what is happening in the general vasculature. Transvaginal color Doppler can therefore be used to assess the effect of HRT on the circulation, and on the uterine arteries in particular.

Tamoxifen and the uterus

It has been proposed that tamoxifen be given to apparently healthy women at increased risk of breast cancer[64]; therefore any deleterious effects it may have on the endometrium are of concern, and it may be necessary to monitor the endometrium of such patients at regular intervals. Tamoxifen has been shown to provide effective treatment for women with all stages of breast cancer. There are also associated physiological benefits that include a fall in circulating cholesterol concentration and the maintenance of bone density in the lumbar spine. However, these benefits derive from the estrogenic action that tamoxifen has on tissues other than the breast. Although other separate mechanisms may be playing a role, it is this possible estrogen agonist activity that has given rise to concern regarding the effect this drug might have on the endometrium.

There have been several reports of the development of endometrial cancer associated with the use of tamoxifen[64–67]. However, the real risk has been hard to evaluate given that both breast and endometrial cancer share both hyperestrogenic and genetic risk factors. In order to evaluate this risk, data from randomized controlled trials are needed[68]. A recent study examined the endometrium of women taking part in a randomized breast cancer prevention trial. The women in the trial received either 20 mg/day of tamoxifen or placebo. Of the women taking tamoxifen, 25% had histological evidence of atypical hyperplasia or polyp formation compared to 4% in the placebo group[69]. In all cases of significant histological abnormality, the endometrial thickness was greater than 8.0 mm and was often cystic in appearance (Figure 13). Furthermore, the uterine artery PI for all polyps and cases of atypical hyperplasia was less than 1.8. In view of the lower dose of drug used in this study it is difficult to ignore this clear evidence of the association between tamoxifen therapy and the development of endometrial lesions. This study suggests that the presence of thick endometrium (≥ 8.0 mm) in women taking tamoxifen is frequently associated with a significant endometrial abnormality, and should be investigated further.

It has also been shown how ultrasound can be used with negative contrast media to demonstrate endometrial lesions associated with the use of tamoxifen therapy[27]. The instillation of sterile saline into the endometrial cavity will help to visualize polyps (Figure 10) that are often difficult to diagnose even with hysteroscopy. In a further study we have repeated scans in women found to have an endometrial thickness of > 8.0 mm on the study described above (n = 80)[70]. Approximately 60% had thick cystic endometrium, and, of these, half had large polyps within the cavity demonstrated by hydrosonography. It is interesting to note that, in this study, outpatient Pipelle sampling failed to get an adequate sample in almost all patients, and missed all of the polyps. These women were then given a 3-month course of sequential progestogen therapy, and it is important to note that the majority failed to have a withdrawal bleed. This suggests that the mechanism of action of tamoxifen on the postmenopausal endometrium is not mediated via its estrogen agonist potential, but by some other mechanism. We believe that ultrasound with hydrosonography is essential for an adequate evaluation of the postmenopausal women taking tamoxifen therapy. Furthermore, the only adequate sampling technique in the presence of abnormal findings is a resected biopsy using a resectoscope.

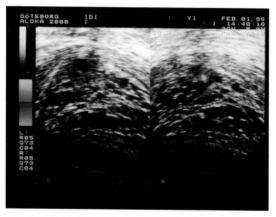

Figure 13 Polypoid–cystic endometrium in a woman taking tamoxifen. Orientation, transducer's tip at the bottom of the figure

THREE-DIMENSIONAL SONOGRAPHY

Since December 1994, the Department of Obstetrics and Gynecology, Sahlgrenska Hospital has had a three-dimensional (3-D) ultrasound scanner (Combison 530, Kretz, Zipf, Austria) in clinical use. A 7.5- or 5-MHz vaginal transducer is used. The volume/region to be examined is located in the B-mode and the volume box, which marks off the region of interest, is set to the appropriate size and position. The 3-D scanning procedure takes 2–8 s depending on the volume box size. Three planes are shown simultaneously on the screen, two of which are realized by the scanning procedure. From these data, the equipment calculates the third plane (Figures 14 and 15). The entire information is held on the work station and can be stored on a changeable hard disk. Further analysis of the different cross-sections can be undertaken and

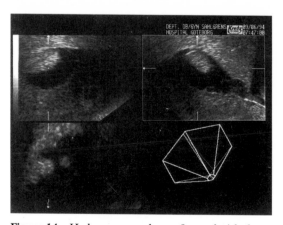

Figure 14 Hydrosonography performed with three-dimensional ultrasound in a woman with an endometrial polyp, shown in three planes

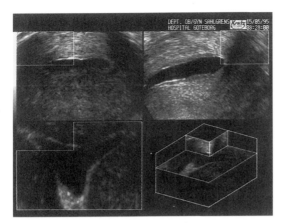

Figure 15 Hydrosonography performed with three-dimensional ultrasound in a woman with a normal endometrial cavity, shown in three planes

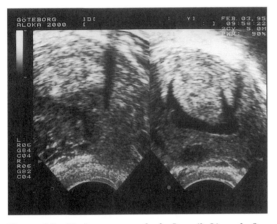

Figure 16 Hydrosonography before (left) and after (right) saline instillation showing a large polyp. Orientation, transducer's tip at the bottom of the figure

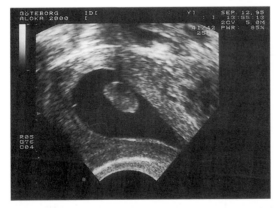

Figure 17 Hydrosonography of an endometrial polyp. Note the regular endometrial cavity. Orientation, transducer's tip at the bottom of the figure

repeated as often as required. In this repeatability lies the advantage of reducing the burden on the patient. It must be emphasized that it is not so much the simultaneous statistical representation of the three planes shown on the screen that helps, but rather, the possibility of 'penetrative/3-D stratification' of an object, facilitated by processing by the work station of a moving object viewed under a simulated fixed light source.

After having performed a couple of thousand 3-D scans, we believe that the feasibility of 3-D methods in the clinical setting using commercially available equipment is imminent. This new technique has some advantages as compared to 2-D ultrasound, such as: new documentation, retrospective analysis in three planes, the patient does not need to be examined for such a long time, and new educational and legal aspects. Furthermore, volume sonography makes possible a new type of volumetry. Hitherto, volumes had to be calculated from distance and surface parameters measured in two dimensions. In 3-D sonography, these measurements can be calculated directly on the volume/region represented.

We also believe that in the future the scanning time will be reduced by 3-D sonography, thus making it more cost-effective as compared to 2-D ultrasound. Standardization of the ultrasound examination is also an option in the future with this equipment.

CONCLUDING REMARKS AND COMMENTS

It is important to be certain that the endometrium has been measured properly. An 'unmeasurable' endometrium should not be accepted as probably being normal. Hydrosonography (Figures 16 and 17) should be performed to try to clarify the situation. If it is still unclear, in symptomatic patients this is an indication for an endometrial biopsy.

Overall, the data reviewed in this chapter suggest that, in the assessment of symptomatic women, an endometrial thickness cut-off level of < 5.0 mm will have a high negative predictive value for the presence of cancer. It must be remembered, however, that this approach to the management of women with postmenopausal bleeding has not yet been subjected to prospective clinical trials.

For women with postmenopausal bleeding, if an endometrial thickness of ≥ 8.0 mm returns a histological diagnosis of atrophy, the possibility of a sampling error should be considered.

There are no data to support the examination of asymptomatic postmenopausal women for the presence of pathology. For a disease of such low incidence, such an approach is unlikely to be fruitful. However, in the 'real' world, given the data from the receiver-operator curves described in the Nordic study, we would perform an outpatient biopsy on an asymptomatic woman not taking hormone replacement therapy, whose endometrium measured more than 8.0 mm.

Women taking HRT have an increased endometrial thickness, and this will change according to the phase of cyclical therapy. In continuous combined regimens, the endometrium is likely to be relatively thin. It is probably best to evaluate such endometria just after the withdrawal bleed. Abnormal bleeding on HRT must still be investigated by biopsy, whilst thick endometrium on HRT is probably just a normal finding in the absence of symptoms. For patients taking tamoxifen therapy, thick endometrium (≥ 8.0 mm) may be associated with the presence of significant endometrial pathology. Of those with thick cystic endometrium, up to 50% will be found to have a polyp following hydrosonography. Conventional outpatient biopsy techniques will fail to detect much of this pathology. We recommend transvaginal ultrasound with hydrosonography for the initial assessment of these women. If a biopsy is needed, a resectoscope may be required.

B-mode ultrasound imaging provides many answers to the evaluation of the pre- and postmenopausal uterus. For example, the endometrial thickness and echogenicity enable the presence or absence of significant pathology to be assessed in the majority of cases. The use of negative contrast agents introduced into the cavity may further enhance diagnostic confidence, and be of particular value in the recognition of polyps.

There are no data that we have seen that demonstrate a practical clinical role for color Doppler in the evaluation of the postmenopausal endometrium.

It is a very valuable research tool, but the addition of color Doppler to B-mode imaging is unnecessary for most gynecologists and radiologists. It adds to the diagnostic picture, but it is not essential. Where color Doppler is of great interest is the study of physiological processes and the effects of exogenous drugs and hormones on blood vessels. In this context, transvaginal color Doppler may act almost as a biological assay of end-organ response[18].

Transvaginal ultrasonography of the endometrium offers a sensitive view to pelvic pathology. The addition of hydrosonography in our view improves diagnostic confidence still further. The limitations are usually related to the operator and so we think that the transvaginal scan should be performed by well-skilled dedicated people. In this way, subtle aspects of pelvic pathology can be detected, and better 'feel' for what is normal and abnormal can be achieved. However, education is the key to the process. Ultrasound is not learned just by sitting in endless lectures collecting CME credits, nor by reading review articles like this. It comes from performing thousands of scans, year in year out, and particularly by comparing your scan findings to your clinical evaluation and then operative experience. From this comes a feeling for what is 'reasonable' in the literature and what is obvious nonsense. In our view, the data suggest a major role for transvaginal ultrasonography in the evaluation of the postmenopausal woman. However, we have concerns with regard to the level of complacency, not so prevalent in obstetric sonography, that seems to exist with regard to training in this area.

Finally, we believe that we have to take the consequences of the TVS findings when scanning the endometrium in women with postmenopausal bleeding, or else the TVS should not be performed. By taking the consequences of the TVS findings, the costs of management strategy of women with postmenopausal bleeding could be reduced by up to 70%, thus making the management of women with postmenopausal bleeding cost-effective[71].

ACKNOWLEDGEMENTS

We would like to thank the Aloka Co. Ltd, (Tokyo, Japan) for the use of their ultrasound equipment. Studies in Göteborg discussed in this chapter were funded in part by the Nordic Cancer Union and the Swedish Medical Research Council. T.H.B. was also funded by the Swedish Medical Research Council.

References

1. Wild, J. and Reid, J. (1957). Progress in techniques of soft tissue examination by 15 Mc pulsed ultrasound. In *Biology and Medicine*, Kelly, E. (ed.) (Washington D.C.: American Institute of Biological Sciences)
2. Kratochwil, A. (1969). Ein neues vaginales Schnittbildverfahren. *Geburtsh. Freuenheilk.*, **29**, 379–85
3. Schwimmer, S. and Lebovic, J. (1984). Transvaginal pelvic ultrasound. *J. Ultrasound Med.*, **3**, 381–3
4. Karlsson, B., Granberg, S., Ridell, B. and Wikland, M. (1994). Endometrial thickness as measured by transvaginal sonography. Interobserver variation. *Ultrasound Obstet. Gynecol.*, **4**, 320–5
5. Cohen, D., Hines, R., Whitman, G. and Plouffe, L. Jr (1993). Ultrasound evaluation of endometrial thickness: how good are the measurements? Abstract. Conjoint meeting of the American Fertility Society and the Canadian Fertility and Andrology Society, Oct 11–14 1993, S140
6. Lehtovirta, P., Cacciatore, B., Wahlström, T. and Ylöstalo, P. (1987). Ultrasonic assessment of endometrial cancer invasion. *J. Clin. Ultrasound*, **15**, 519–24
7. Cacciatore, B., Lehtovirta, P., Wahlström, T., Ylänen, K. and Ylöstalo, P. (1989). Contribution of vaginal scanning to sonographic evaluation of endometrial cancer invasion. *Acta Scand. Oncol.*, **28**, 585–8
8. Fleischer, A., Dudley, B., Entman, S., Baxter, J., Kalameris, G. and Everette, J. Jr (1987). Myometrial invasion: sonographic assessment. *Radiology*, **162**, 307–10
9. Auslender, R., Bornstein, J., Dirnfeld, M., Kogan, O., Atad, J. and Abramovici, H. (1993). Vaginal ultrasonography in patients with postmenopausal bleeding. *Ultrasound Obstet. Gynecol.*, **3**, 426–8
10. Bakos, O., Smith, P. and Heimer, G. (1994). Transvaginal ultrasonography for identifying endometrial pathology in postmenopausal women. Thesis, Uppsala, Sweden
11. Nasri, M. and Coast, G. (1989). Correlation of ultrasound findings and endometrial histopathology in postmenopausal women. *Br. J. Obstet. Gynaecol.*, **96**, 1333–8
12. Grimes, D. (1982). Dilatation and curettage: a reappraisal. *Am. J. Obstet. Gynecol.*, **142**, 1–6
13. Vuopala, S. (1977). Diagnostic accuracy and clinical applicability of cytological and histological methods for investigating endometrial carcinoma. *Acta Obstet. Gynecol. Scand.*, (Suppl.), **70**, 22–5
14. MacKenzie, I. and Bibby, J. (1978). Critical assessment of dilatation and curettage in 1029 women. *Lancet*, **2**, 566–8
15. Nasri, M., Shepherd, J., Setchell, M., Lowe, D. and Chard, T. (1991). Sonographic depiction of postmenopausal endometrium with transabdominal and transvaginal scanning. *Ultrasound Obstet. Gynecol.*, **1**, 279–83
16. Holst, J., Koskela, O. and von Schoultz, B. (1983). Endometrial findings following curettage in 2018 women according to age and indications. *Annales Chirurg. Gynaecol.*, **72**, 274–7
17. Lidor, A., Ismajovich, B., Confino, E. and David, M. (1986). Histopathological findings in 226 women with post-menopausal uterine bleeding. *Acta Obstet. Gynecol. Scand.*, **65**, 41–3
18. Word, B., Gravlee, C. and Wideman, G. (1958). The fallacy of simple uterine curettage. *Obstet. Gynecol.*, **12**, 642–8
19. Stock, R. and Kanbour, A. (1975). Prehysterectomy curettage. *Obstet. Gynecol.*, **45**, 537–41
20. Koonings, P., Moyer, D. and Grimes, D. (1990). A randomized clinical trial comparing Pipelle and Tis-U-Trap for endometrial biopsy. *Obstet. Gynecol.*, **75**, 293–5
21. Stovall, T., Solomon, S. and Ling, F. (1989). Endometrial sampling prior to hysterectomy. *Obstet. Gynecol.*, **73**, 405–9
22. Karlsson, B., Granberg, S., Wikland, M., Ryd, W. and Norström, A. (1993). Endovaginal scanning of the endometrium compared to cytology and

histology in women with postmenopausal bleeding. *Gynecol. Oncol.*, **50**, 173–8

23. Gimpleson, R. and Rappold, H.(1988). A comparative study between panoramic hysteroscopy with directed biopsies and dilatation and curettage. *Am. J. Obstet. Gynecol.*, **158**, 489–92

24. Townsend, D., Fields, G., McCausland, A. and Kauffman, K. (1993). Diagnostic and operative hysteroscopy in the management of persistent postmenopausal bleeding. *Obstet. Gynecol.*, **82**, 419–21

25. Parsons, A. K. and Lense, J. J. (1993). Sonohysterography for endometrial abnormalities: preliminary results. *J. Clin. Ultrasound.*, **21**, 87–95

26. Goldstein, S. (1994). Use of ultrasonography for triage of perimenopausal patients with unexplained uterine bleeding. *Am. J. Obstet. Gynecol.*, **170**, 565–70

27. Bourne, T. H., Lawton, F., Leather, A., Granberg, S., Campbell, S. and Collins, W. P. (1994). Use of intracavitary saline instillation and transvaginal ultrasonography to detect tamoxifen-associated endometrial polyps. *Ultrasound Obstet. Gynecol.*, **4**, 73–5

28. Osmers, R., Völksen, M. and Schauer, A. (1990). Vaginosonography for early detection of endometrial carcinoma? *Lancet*, **335**, 1569–71

29. Granberg, S., Friberg, L.-G., Norström, A. and Wikland, M. (1988). Endovaginal ultrasound scanning of women with postmenopausal bleeding. *J. Ultrasound Med.*, **7**:(s.10), 283

30. Sheth, S., Hamper, U. and Kurman, R. (1993). Thickened endometrium in the postmenopausal woman: sonographic–pathological correlation. *Radiology*, **187**, 135–9

31. Botsis, D., Kassanos, D., Pyrgiotis, E. and Zourlas, P. (1992). Vaginosonography of the endometrium in postmenopausal women. *Clin. Exp. Obstet. Gynecol.*, **19**, 189–92

32. Dörum, A., Kristensen, B., Langebrekke, A., Sörnes, T. and Skaar, O. (1993). Evaluation of endometrial thickness measured by endovaginal ultrasound in women with postmenopausal bleeding. *Acta Obstet. Gynecol. Scand.*, **72**, 116–19

33. Karlsson, B., Granberg, S., Wikland, M. Ylöstalo, P., Kiserud, T. and Marsal, K. (1995). Transvaginal sonography of the endometrium in postmenopausal women to identify endometrial abnormality – a Nordic multi-center study. *Am. J. Obstet. Gynecol.*, **172**, 1488–94

34. Granberg, S., Wikland, M., Karlsson, B., Norström, A. and Friberg, L-G. (1991). Endometrial thickness as measured by endovaginal ultrasound for identifying endometrial abnormality. *Am. J. Obstet. Gynecol.*, **164**, 47–52

35. Fleischer, A., Kalemeris, G., Machin, J., Entmann, S. S. and James, E. (1986). Sonographic depiction of normal and abnormal endometrium with histopathological correlation. *J. Ultrasound Med.*, **5**, 445–52

36. Fleischer, A., Gordon, A., Entman, S. and Kepple, D. (1990). Transvaginal scanning of the endometrium. *J. Clin. Ultrasound*, **18**, 337–49

37. Varner, R., Sparks, J., Cameron, C., Roberts, L. and Soong, S.-J. (1991). Transvaginal sonography of the endometrium in postmenopausal women. *Obstet. Gynecol.*, **78**, 195–9

38. Bourne, T. H., Campbell, S., Whitehead, M., Royston, P., Steer, C. and Collins, W. (1990). Detection of endometrial cancer in postmenopausal women by transvaginal ultrasonography and color flow imaging. *Br. Med. J.*, **301**, 369–70

39. Rudelstorfer, R., Nanz, S. and Bernaschek, G. (1990). Vaginosonography and its diagnostic value in patients with postmenopausal bleeding. *Arch. Gynecol. Obstet.*, **248**, 37–44

40. Goldstein, S., Nachtigall, M., Snyder, J. and Nachtigall, L. (1990). Endometrial assessment by vaginal ultrasonography before endometrial sampling in patients with postmenopausal bleeding. *Am. J. Obstet. Gynecol.*, **163**, 119–23

41. Abu Hmeidan, F., Bilek, K., Baier, D., Nuwayhid, M. and Kade, R. (1992). Das sonographische Bild des Endometriumkarzinomas. *Ultraschall. in Med.*, **13**, 178–82

42. Weiner, Z., Beck, D., Rottem, S., Brandes, J. and Thaler, I. (1993). Uterine artery flow velocity waveforms and color flow imaging in women with perimenopausal and postmenopausal bleeding. *Acta Obstet. Gynecol. Scand.*, **72**, 162–6

43. Ferrazzi, E., Torri, V., Trio, D., Zannoni, E., Severi, F. and Dordoni, D. (1996). Transvaginal sonographic endometrial thickness: a useful test to predict atrophy in menopausal bleeding: an Italian multicenter trial. *Ultrasound Obstet. Gynecol.*, **7**, 315–21

44. Carlson, J., Arger, P., Thompson, S. and Carlson, E. (1991). Clinical and pathologic correlation of endometrial cavity fluid detected by ultrasound in the postmenopausal patient. *Obstet. Gynecol.*, **77**, 119–22

45. Gull, B., Karlsson, B., Milsom, I., Wikland, M. and Granberg, S. (1995). Uterine cavity fluid – possible causes in a representative sample of asymptomatic PM-women compared with a matched control group. *Ultrasound Obstet. Gynecol.*, **6**, 111–12

46. Steer, C. W., Campbell, S., Pampligione, J., Kingsland, C. R., Mason, B. A. and Collins, W. P. (1990). Transvaginal colour flow imaging of the uterine arteries during the ovarian and menstrual cycles. *Hum. Reprod.*, **5**, 391

47. Bourne, T. H., Hillard, T., Whitehead, M. I., Crook, D. and Campbell, S. (1990). Evidence for a rapid effect of oestrogens on the arterial

status of postmenopausal women. *Lancet*, **335**, 1470–1

48. Bourne, T. H., Campbell, S., Steer, C., Royston, P., Whitehead, M. and Collins, W. (1991). Detection of endometrial cancer by transvaginal ultrasonography with color flow imaging and blood flow analysis: a preliminary report. *Gynecol. Oncol.*, **40**, 253–9

49. Kurjak, A., Zalud, I., Jurkovic, D., Alfirovic, Z. and Miljan, M. (1989). Transvaginal color flow Doppler for the assessment of pelvic circulation. *Acta Obstet. Gynecol. Scand.*, **68**, 131–5

50. Hata, K., Makihara, K., Hata, T., Takahashi, K. and Kitao, M. (1991). Transvaginal color Doppler imaging for haemodynamic assessment of tumors in the reproductive tract. *Int. J. Gynecol. Obstet.*, **44**, 306–11

51. Kurjak, A. and Zalud, I. (1991). The characterisation of uterine tumors by transvaginal colour Doppler. *Ultrasound Obstet. Gynecol.*, **1**, 50–2

52. Creighton, S., Bourne, T. H., Lawton, F., Crayford, T. J. B., Vyas, S., Campbell, S. and Collins, W. P. (1994). Use of transvaginal ultrasonography with color Doppler imaging to determine an appropriate treatment regimen for uterine fibroids with a GnRH agonist before surgery: a preliminary study. *Ultrasound Obstet. Gynecol.*, **4**, 494–8

53. Bourne, T. H., Crayford, T., Hampson, J., Collins, W. P. and Campbell, S. (1992). The detection of endometrial cancer by transvaginal ultrasonography with colour Doppler. *Ultrasound Obstet. Gynecol.*, **2**, 75

54. Ylöstalo, P., Granberg, S., Bäckström, A-C. and Hirsjärvi-Lahti, T. (1996). Uterine findings by transvaginal sonography during percutaneous estrogen treatment in postmenopausal women. *Maturitas*, **23**, 313–17

55. Gull, B., Karlsson, B., Milsom, I., Wikland, M. and Granberg, S. (1996). Transvaginal sonography of the endometrium in a representative sample of postmenopausal women. *Ultrasound Obstet. Gynecol.*, **7**, 322–7

56. Lin, M., Gosik, B., Wolf, S. and Feldesman, M. (1991). Endometrial thickness after menopause: effect of hormone replacement. *Radiology*, **180**, 427–32

57. Meuvissen, J., van Langen, H., Moret, E. and Navarro-Morquecho, I. (1992). Monitoring of estrogen replacement therapy by vaginosonography of the endometrium. *Maturitas*, **15**, 33–7

58. Levine, D., Gosink, B. and Johnson, L. (1995). Change in endometrial thickness in postmenopausal women undergoing hormone replacement therapy. *Radiology*, **197**, 603–8

59. Padwick, M. L., Whitehead, M. I., Coffer, A. and King, R. J. B. (1989). Demonstration of estrogen receptor related protein in female tissues. In

Studd, J. W. W., Whitehead, M. I. (eds.) *The Menopause*, pp. 227–33. (Oxford: Blackwell)

60. Hillard, T. C., Bourne, T. H., Crayford, T., Collins, W. P., Campbell, S. and Whitehead, M. I. (1992). Differential effects of transdermal estradiol and sequential progestagens on impendance to flow within the uterine arteries of postmenopausal women. *Fertil. Steril.*, **58**, 959–63

61. Marsh, M. S., Bourne, T. H., Whitehead, M. I., Collins, W. P. and Campbell, S. (1994). The temporal effect of progesterone on uterine artery pulsatility index in postmenopausal women receiving sequential hormone replacement therapy. *Fertil. Steril.*, **62**, 771–4

62. de Ziegler, D., Bessis, R. and Frydman, R. (1991). Vascular resistance of uterine arteries: physiological effects of estradiol and progesterone. *Fertil. Steril.*, **55**, 775–7

63. Pines, A., Fishman, E. Z., Levo, Y., Averbuch, M., Lidor, A., Drory, Y., Finkelstein, A., Hetman-Peri, M., Moshkowitz, M., Ben-Ari, E. and Ayalon, D. (1991). The effects of hormone replacement therapy in normal postmenopausal women: measurements of Doppler-derived parameters of aortic flow. *Am. J. Obstet. Gynecol.*, **164**, 806–12

64. Powles, T. J., Hardy, S. E., Ashley, S. E., Farrington, G. M., Cosgrove, D., Davey, J. B., Dowsett, M., McKinna, J. A., Nash, A. G., Sinnett, H. D., Tillyer, C. R. and Treleaven, J. G. (1989). A pilot trial to evaluate the acute toxicity and feasibility of tamoxifen for prevention of breast cancer. *Br. J. Cancer*, **60**, 126–31

65. Cohen, I. (1993). Endometrial changes in postmenopausal women treated with tamoxifen for breast cancer. *Br. J. Obstet. Gynaecol.*, **100**, 567–70

66. Fornander, T. (1989). Adjuvant tamoxifen therapy in early breast cancer: occurrence of new primary cancers. *Lancet*, **1**, 117–20

67. Neven, P. (1993). Tamoxifen and endometrial lesions. *Lancet*, **2**, 452

68. Craig Jordon, V. (1993). How safe is tamoxifen? Only randomized controlled trials can decide. *Br. Med. J.*, **307**, 1371–2

69. Kedar, R. P., Bourne, T. H., Powles, T. J., Collins, W. P., Cosgrove, D. O. and Campbell, S. (1994). Effects of tamoxifen on the uterus and ovaries of women involved in a randomized breast cancer prevention trial. *Lancet*, **343**, 34–8

70. Bourne, T. H., Grubock, K., Athanasiou, S., Powles, T., Campbell, S., Cosgrove, D. and Collis, W. P. (1994). The use of ultrasound to study the effects of tamoxifen on the uterus of postmenopausal women. *Ultrasound Obstet. Gynecol.*, **4** S1, 131

71. Granberg, M. and Granberg, S. (1996). Cost-effectiveness in the management of women with postmenopausal bleeding. *Acta Scand. Gynecol.*, in press

Transvaginal sonography of the endometrium in postmenopausal breast cancer patients receiving tamoxifen

5

C. Exacoustòs, D. Arduini and C. Romanini

INTRODUCTION

Tamoxifen is usually classified as an estrogen antagonist as it competes with estrogens for estrogen receptors (ER). Its main use since the early 1970s has been in the treatment of advanced breast cancer and in the course of time it has become the endocrine treatment of choice for all stages of breast cancer in postmenopausal patients with positive ER. An overview analysis of the effectiveness of adjuvant tamoxifen treatment for breast cancer shows that tamoxifen does confer an absolute survival benefit[1–4]. The preservation of bone mineral density and lowered cholesterol observed in tamoxifen-treated postmenopausal women is thought to have additional possible benefits to the decreased prevalence of contralateral breast cancer. These findings were used as the clinical rationale for current trials exploring the use of tamoxifen as a chemoprevention agent in healthy women at high risk of developing breast cancer[2,3,5–7].

The use of tamoxifen for the prevention of breast cancer is not without controversy because of its carcinogenic potential.

TAMOXIFEN: MECHANISMS OF ACTION AND EFFECTS

Tamoxifen is thought to inhibit breast cancer growth by competitively blocking ER, thereby inhibiting estrogen-induced growth.

Tamoxifen inhibits the production of the estrogen-stimulated growth factor, transforming growth factor-α (TGF-α), and by blocking the estrogen action increases the production of some members of the TGF-β family that are known inhibitors of epithelial cell growth. Furthermore, tamoxifen may block the action of stimulatory paracrine growth factors on ER-positive cells and reduce the availability of insulin-like growth factors 1 (IGF-1) both in the circulation and locally in the tissues. These effects of tamoxifen could reduce the growth of both ER-positive and ER-negative disease[2]. Tamoxifen acts therefore primarily by suppressing the growth of breast cancer rather than by causing cell death, which indicates that treatment with adjuvant tamoxifen achieves optimal results only if it is administered for an extended period of time[1,2,8]. Recently a review conducted by members of the National Surgical Adjuvant Breast and Bowel Project (NSABP) in Pittsburgh found that there is no advantage in taking tamoxifen for more than 5 years, perhaps because the tumors exposed to the drug for long periods adapt and begin responding to it as they do to estrogen[9,10].

Tamoxifen is usually regarded as a safe drug, but its administration for long time periods warrants a much more critical look at possible adverse reactions. The side-effects of tamoxifen that are most commonly cited include hot flushes, nausea, vomiting and vaginal dryness or vaginitis, and more serious but rare complications are thromboembolic events and hyperlipidemia[3]. The side-effects that develop during long-term administration become a concern. Perhaps the deepest concern is the carcinogenic potential of tamoxifen since it is a proven carcinogen in the rat. Tamoxifen itself is not genotoxic but is activated by cytochrome P450, the drug-metabolizing enzyme, to form reactive intermediates that bind covalently to DNA to create adducts and carcinogenic risk[11]. Tamoxifen is converted to several metabolites, most of which are antiestrogens, but can act as weak partial agonists in the absence of estradiol[2,8]. It has been shown that tamoxifen has different agonistic, antagonistic, or carcinogenic properties depending on the animal species examined. In chickens, it acts as an estrogen antagonist, in mice as a pure estrogen agonist and in rats can cause cancers in the liver, but not in other tissues[11]. Gottardis and co-workers[12] showed that tamoxifen induced a reduction in cell numbers in a breast cancer and stimulated cell growth in an endometrial cancer after both tumors were transplanted into the same animal. Therefore, since tamoxifen has a species-specific and tissue-specific action, quantitative prediction from experimental data of any human risk, in any tissue, is not possible.

Hormone promotion may also be important in other tissues such as those of the ovary, liver, eye, bone and vessels with positive or negative side-effects.

The possible synergism of genotoxicity and estrogenic promotion by tamoxifen makes the uterus a primary site of potential carcinogenic risk in humans. Other organs potentially at special risk in humans are those with a high cellular proliferation rate, such as bone marrow and those tissues that may be exposed to high levels of carcinogenic metabolites such as liver, stomach and colon[11,13-15]. The available data on tamoxifen and cancer of the gastrointestinal tract and the liver suggest that tamoxifen could be carcinogenic in humans but not that it *is* carcinogenic. This preliminary information has to be now essentially evaluated by methodical clinical trials similar to the approach that has been taken for the association of endometrial cancer and tamoxifen.

TAMOXIFEN: EFFECTS ON THE ENDOMETRIUM

Although the effects of tamoxifen on the endometrium have been widely studied[3,5-7,14-35], they are not fully understood. They do, however, appear to depend on the menopausal status of the patient.

In premenopausal women, tamoxifen induces hyperestrogenemia by increasing serum estrogen level[36,37]. High levels of estradiol may antagonize the receptor-blocking effect of tamoxifen, and this may produce a situation in which breast tumor proliferation might be promoted and not inhibited. Tamoxifen seems therefore to be less effective in premenopausal breast cancer women, probably also in relation to lower ER expression by the cancer[27]. Premenopausal women taking tamoxifen may have irregular periods or develop amenorrhea, but most continue to have normal menstrual cycles. Premenopausal women on tamoxifen therapy could be at elevated risk for ovarian cancer[32] and ovarian cysts due to the elevated estrogen stimulation[6,29].

In postmenopausal women, tamoxifen acts as an antiestrogen on breast cancer cells and as a weak estrogen on the uterus and a large spectrum of pathological uterine findings have been recognized with long-term tamoxifen therapy.

Several studies[20,24-29,33-35] have reported an association between tamoxifen therapy and proliferative endometrium or endometrial hyperplasia in postmenopausal patients. Endocervical and endometrial polyps have been also consistently found in patients receiving tamoxifen. Most of these polyps show mildly hyperplastic changes with secretory glands or atrophic dilated cystic glands with round contours.

A number of authors have reported that, because of its estrogenic agonist function on the endometrium, tamoxifen can induce the development of endometrial cancer[17,33]. Fonander and colleagues[18], in a study of 1800 postmenopausal women, found 13 new endometrial adenocarcinomas in the tamoxifen-treated group compared to the control group. In their interesting studies, the groups of Lahti[26], Neven[8], Cohen[20,29] and Van Leeuwen[30] observed only a few cases of endometrial cancer, not sufficient to demonstrate a clear relationship between tamoxifen and endometrial cancer. No endometrial cancer was found among 1070 postmenopausal women in the

Scottish trial[16] on tamoxifen. Recently the Stockholm trial, which analyzed 2729 breast cancer patients of whom 1372 were on tamoxifen therapy, observed a nearly sixfold increase in endometrial cancer among the tamoxifen-treated patients with a relative risk of 4.1[14]. Also the data obtained in the National Adjuvant Breast and Bowel Project revealed an increase in endometrial cancer in long-term tamoxifen-treated patients with a relative risk of 7.5[38]. On the other hand, some authors[32,33] recently reported a low risk for endometrial cancer in patients treated for less than 2 years, always associated with a decreased risk of contralateral breast cancer. The true incidence of endometrial cancer related to tamoxifen is difficult to estimate from all these studies, also considering that different dosages of tamoxifen were used.

Some authors have reported that patients receiving tamoxifen develop high-grade carcinomas[22,23], but in general the endometrial cancers described in the literature associated with tamoxifen do not differ in grade from carcinomas that occur in patients not receiving this hormone.

With the knowledge available today, it appears prudent to recommend close follow-up of patients receiving tamoxifen in order to identify possible side-effects of this therapy on the endometrium.

TAMOXIFEN: TRANSVAGINAL SONOGRAPHIC ENDOMETRIAL FINDINGS

Transvaginal ultrasound has been proposed as an accurate, simple, non-invasive and painless method for the examination of the endometrium in postmenopausal women[39–45]. Recently, transvaginal color flow Doppler has been suggested as a screening method for endometrial cancer[46–50]. Nevertheless, the best methods for the diagnosis of endometrial lesions are invasive. Hysteroscopy has been found to be more accurate than other invasive endometrial diagnostic methods, especially for focal lesions and polyps[8,51–54], but histological evaluation remains the gold standard of any endometrial examination.

There are a lot of studies[5,20,26,29,55–62] which describe the various endometrial patterns observed by transvaginal ultrasound in patients receiving tamoxifen and the histological findings associated with these patterns. The results differ widely, particularly in the presence of endometrial pathology in these patients.

Only a few[26,55,56,62] of these studies compared sonographic findings and hysteroscopy. Most of them used blind sample methods, like endometrial cytology or dilatation and curettage, to detect endometrial lesions, but these are not as accurate as hysteroscopy with guided biopsy. The use of blind methods for endometrial evaluation can, for example, miss polyps because curettage or sampling of the surface of the polyp may give a histological diagnosis of atrophic endometrium. Therefore the prevalence of endometrial pathology may be underestimated because focal endometrial lesions are difficult to detect by these conventional techniques. This may explain some of the disparities seen in apparent disease prevalence reported in the literature in patients on tamoxifen therapy.

On the basis of blind endometrial sampling alone, which often gives insufficient material for histological analysis, many authors[5,20,25,29,63] have reported in patients receiving tamoxifen a histological diagnosis of atrophic endometrium associated with thickened endometrial sonographic pattern with small cystic areas. Hysteroscopy, and recently sonohysterography (transvaginal sonography with instillation of intracavitary saline), has been proposed to improve the diagnosis of endometrial polyps in patients receiving tamoxifen.

Other authors[59,60] have observed a histological and hysteroscopic atrophic endometrium associated with an echographic and sonohysteroscopic view of a thickened endometrium with cystic areas in the subendometrial space. These findings can be explained by a histology pattern of atrophic endometrium with dilated cystic glands which are lined with low columnar epithelium or with adenomyosal foci forming microcysts in the proximal myometrium. The cystic change seen in the atrophic glands in hysterectomy specimens of tamoxifen patients is often not observed in biopsies because tissue fragmentation from the procedures disrupts the glands[64]. This could be the reason why histological findings of atrophic endometrium are sometimes associated with a sonographic finding of thickened endometrium with cystic areas[60]. One of the problems met with in assessing patients receiving tamoxifen is that outpatient biopsy techniques provide inadequate samples in this specific group of patients[29], therefore the hysteroscopic or sonohysterographic view of the uterine cavity becomes diagnostic in the case of cystic atrophic endometrium or of endometrial polyps.

An analysis[62] of endometrial echotexture in postmenopausal patients receiving 20–30 mg daily of tamoxifen for at least 12 months demonstrated four different sonographic patterns:

(1) An echogenic endometrium with regular borders, integrity of the subendometrial halo and homogeneous echotexture;

(2) An echogenic endometrium with regular borders containing small anechoic cysts (Figure 1);

(3) An echogenic endometrium with inhomogeneous echotexture sometimes with small cystic areas, irregular borders and integrity of the subendometrial halo (Figure 2); and

(4) An echogenic endometrium with inhomogeneous echotexture, irregular borders and interrupted subendometrial halo (Figure 3).

The presence of intracavitary fluid was also observed in some cases but always with a minimal fluid volume (less than the thickness of one layer of the endometrium)[48].

These various patterns have been correlated with hysteroscopic and histological findings[62]. The first endometrial pattern is often associated

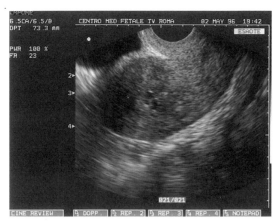

Figure 2 Transvaginal sonographic view of a thickened endometrium with irregular border and small anechoic cystic areas: an endometrial cystic atrophy in a postmenopausal patient receiving tamoxifen

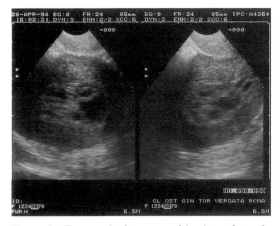

Figure 1 Transvaginal sonographic view of a polypoid endometrial pattern with regular border and small anechoic cystic areas: an endometrial polyp in a postmenopausal patient receiving tamoxifen

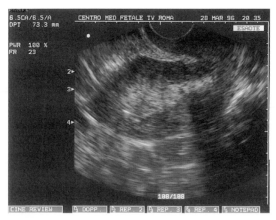

Figure 3 Transvaginal sonographic view of a thickened endometrium with irregular border and hyperechoic inhomogeneous echotexture: an endometrial cancer in a postmenopausal patient receiving tamoxifen

with a regular atrophic postmenopausal endometrium or a weak proliferative regular endometrium; the second with polyps filling the uterine cavity, often surrounded by a thin atrophic endometrium resulting in a sonographic view of thickened endometrium with regular borders (Figure 1). Histology often reveals within these polyps a cystic glandular hyperplasia or dilated cystic glands lined with atrophic endometrium[61,62]. These histological findings could explain the sonographic view of small cystic areas within the endometrium which are sometimes defined as polypoid[62] or honeycombed[65]. Most of these polyps show histologically a dense fibrotic stroma[61,64], but some authors have reported stroma with decidual changes that could not be attributed to any exogenous progestin use[29,58,65].

The third sonographic pattern is seen in the presence of a hysteroscopically thickened endometrium with a regular or irregular surface due to the presence of dilated cystic glands (Figure 2). In this pattern, hysteroscopy does not always allow an endometrial biopsy and, when endometrial samples are obtained, an atrophic or a weakly proliferative endometrium is histologically reported. Endometrial hyperplasia and cancer are always associated with pattern 4 (Figure 3). Comparing endometrial thickness to the various endometrial sonographic patterns, it has been observed that patterns 1 and 3 have a width which is always less than 12 mm, that polypoid pattern and polyps are observed with a thickness of more than 6 mm and that an endometrial pattern less than 5 mm is always associated (as in postmenopausal patients not receiving tamoxifen) with endometrial atrophy. It can happen that pattern 3 is associated with polyps and, in these cases, a regular border cannot be observed, but polyps can be suspected when there is a greater endometrial thickness. Sonohysterography could be helpful in diagnosing this endometrial pathology (Figure 4).

These results suggest[26,29,62,65,66] that all postmenopausal women receiving tamoxifen, with an endometrial thickness > 5 mm, should undergo hysteroscopy and/or endometrial biopsy.

So far we ourselves have managed 102 patients receiving tamoxifen; of these 96 were postmenopausal and six premenopausal. Two of the 96 postmenopausal patients were hysterectomized and had an ovarian cyst. Of the 94 non-hysterectomized patients, 75 were asymptomatic and 19 had vaginal bleeding. The endometrial thickness distribution (Figure 5) shows that only 11% of patients receiving tamoxifen had a width ≤ 5 mm and that 51% had a thickness > 10 mm.

The mean endometrial thickness of asymptomatic patients was significantly lower (11.1 ± 5.7 mm) than in patients with vaginal bleeding (16.1 ± 7.7 mm), and only one patient with bleeding had an endometrial width ≤ 5 mm.

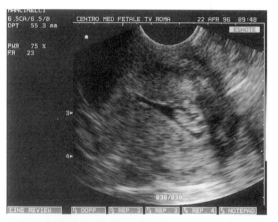

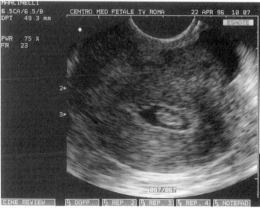

Figure 4 Transvaginal sonographic views (upper panel, sagittal; lower panel, short axis) of an endometrial polyp and thickened endometrium after intracavitary fluid instillation in a postmenopausal patient receiving tamoxifen; note the small anechoic cystic areas within the polyp and endometrium

The hysteroscopic and histological findings obtained in asymptomatic women and patients with vaginal bleeding are reported in Table 1. A high percentage of polyps (40%), two endometrial cancers in patients with bleeding and one atypical hyperplasia in an asymptomatic patient were detected.

Endometrial thickness in the presence of polyps was always more than 6 mm, and, when hyperplasia and cancer were detected, was more than 8 mm. Our data, like those of other authors[29,39], show how the application of cut-off values for endometrial thickness derived from the general population may not be applied to this specific group of women. Higher cut-off values for endometrial thickness (8 or 10 mm) have been proposed by other authors[34,39] in order to restrict invasive diagnostic methods to

those cases in which there is a strong suspicion of endometrial pathology. Nevertheless, in patients taking tamoxifen, we still use a cut-off for endometrial width of 5 mm, considering these patients at high risk for endometrial lesions, especially in the presence of vaginal bleeding. Data from randomized large controlled trials are needed to determine when and how to manage asymptomatic women with a thick endometrium who are receiving tamoxifen.

A high incidence of polyps of 10–20% has also been reported by several authors[5,8,20,29,57,60,66,67] and it is peculiar that these polyps induced by tamoxifen treatment all had a typical polypoid or honeycombed endometrial pattern on sonography. Only the few studies[26,55,62] that use hysteroscopy or sonohysterography as a diagnostic method show a higher percentage of polyps (30–40%), confirming the fact that with blind endometrial sampling polyps could be difficult to detect.

A correlation between endometrial thickness and duration of tamoxifen treatment or cumulative dose of tamoxifen has been observed by some authors but not confirmed by others[25].

A correlation of hysteroscopic/histological findings with the postmenopausal period of start of tamoxifen treatment suggests that there is a greater induction of endometrial growth when the treatment is started many years after menopause. In patients who start the therapy only a

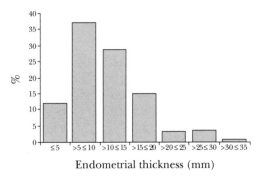

Figure 5 Distribution of endometrial thickness in postmenopausal patients receiving tamoxifen

Table 1 Hysteroscopic and histological findings in non-hysterectomized postmenopausal patients receiving tamoxifen

	Asymptomatic (n = 75)				Vaginal bleeding (n = 19)				Total (n = 94)
	n	Mean ± SD	Minimum	Maximum	n	Mean ± SD	Minimim	Maximum	
Endometrial thickness > 5 mm	65				18				83
Hysteroscopies performed in outpatients	54				18				72
Hysteroscopic/histological findings									
Cancer	0				2	17.0 ± 8.5	11	23	3
Complex hyperplasia	2	13.9 ± 2.8	11	15	0				2
Simple hyperplasia	11	11.6 ± 2.4	9	15	4	14.2 ± 6.6	10	15	15
Polyp	28	13.6 ± 6.0	7	26	11	19.3 ± 7.6	8	31	39
Atrophy	13	10.4 ± 4.2	6	12	1	6.0			14

fews years after the menopause the estrogenic effects on the endometrium seem to be very slight and an atrophic endometrium can often be observed. This can be explained by the different estrogenic effects of tamoxifen depending on the estradiol concentration[2,8]. At low concentrations of estradiol there is a weak estrogenic effect; with increasing estradiol concentrations tamoxifen antagonizes growth; at high estradiol concentrations the inhibitory effect is reversed and growth is again stimulated[1-3,8]. In the postmenopausal period, particularly many years after menopause, the circulating levels of estradiol are very low and tamoxifen acts as a weak estrogen. At the beginning of menopause there is still some circulating estradiol and this can be probably related to the lesser response to tamoxifen of postmenopausal women who start the treatment only a short time after menopause.

Hence an accurate transvaginal monitoring of postmenopausal breast cancer patients receiving tamoxifen has been suggested, particularly in those who start therapy many years after the onset of menopause, in order to identify women at risk who necessitate further invasive diagnostic methods.

TAMOXIFEN: TRANSVAGINAL SONOGRAPHIC COLOR FLOW DOPPLER FINDINGS

Although the sonographic endometrial morphology in patients receiving tamoxifen has been widely described, there are only a few studies which analyze the effects of tamoxifen on uterine blood flow[5,62,63,65-67].

The color flow Doppler examination has demonstrated a uterine artery blood flow impedance [as reflected by the pulsatility index (PI) and resistance index (RI)] that is significantly lower in tamoxifen-treated patients compared to untreated controls[5,62,63,65-67]. The blood velocity changes due to vasodilatation are very similar to those described in postmenopausal women receiving estrogen replacement therapy[68-70].

No correlation has been found between endometrial sonographic widths and uterine PI[62,63,65] (Figure 6). This means that the PI value

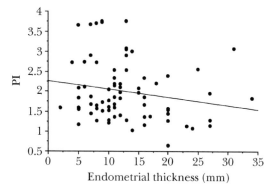

Figure 6 Correlation between endometrial thickness and uterine artery pulsatility index (PI) in postmenopausal patients receiving tamoxifen ($y = -0.021x + 2.3$; $r^2 = 0.034$; $p = 0.1133$)

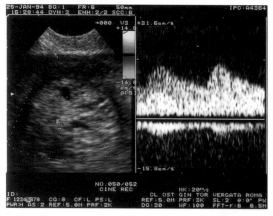

Figure 7 Transvaginal color and pulsed Doppler findings in a postmenopausal patient with an endometrial polyp receiving tamoxifen. Waveform analysis of an artery within the polyp shows low resistance and high diastolic frequencies

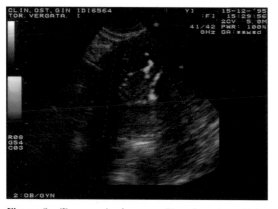

Figure 8 Transvaginal power Doppler view of the vascularization in an endometrial cancer in a postmenopausal patient receiving tamoxifen

is not always lower in patients with pathological endometrial conditions as compared to those without any endometrial lesions. Although the correlation between uterine artery blood flow parameters and hysteroscopic/histological findings shows a tendency towards lower impedance in patients with polyps, hyperplasia and cancer compared to patients with atrophic endometrium receiving tamoxifen[65], the PI values in patients with atrophic endometrium are lower in tamoxifen-treated than in untreated women. These data suggest that the estrogenic action of tamoxifen on uterine vessels may be independent of endometrial growth, which can be explained by the hypothesis that tamoxifen may be organ-specific, confirming that the response to tamoxifen is different for different tissues.

Lower impedance to flow has also been observed[62,66,70] in endometrial and subendometrial vessels, and reflected by an increased diastolic frequency with very low RI (Figure 7).

Since pulsed Doppler flow sonography appears to contribute to the diagnosis of endometrial cancer in postmenopausal patients by detecting low RI in the uterine arteries and in the arteries within the tumor[46–50,71–73] attempts to apply the same criteria to tamoxifen patients have been made. No difference between malignant and benign endometrial pathology based on color Doppler sonography in patients receiving tamoxifen has been established since all these studies had too few cases of endometrial cancer to conclude that pulsed Doppler flow is probably not useful in distinguishing benign from malignant endometrial pathology in these patients[65,66]. However, low uterine and endometrial artery RI in patients receiving tamoxifen are very similar to those of patients with endometrial cancer not receiving tamoxifen[71–73]. Differences between benign and malignant endometrial pathology by color Doppler in

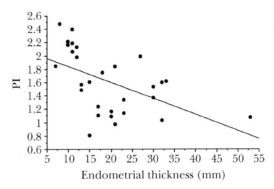

Figure 9 Correlation between endometrial thickness and uterine artery pulsatility index (PI) in postmenopausal patients with endometrial cancer *not* receiving tamoxifen ($y = -0.024x + 2.1$; $r^2 = 0.3$; $p = 0.0039$)

tamoxifen-treated patients are perhaps better revealed by vascular distribution than by the impedance indexes[35]. Atrophic endometria are often avascular, and in benign polyps usually only a few regular vessels are seen (Figure 7); otherwise in cancer an abundant irregular vascularization can be observed (Figure 8).

Furthermore, in patients with endometrial cancer not receiving tamoxifen, we have observed a significant correlation between endometrial thickness and uterine artery PI value, suggesting that uterine resistance may be dependent on tumor volume (Figure 9). This relationship cannot be observed in patients receiving tamoxifen because low uterine impedance is caused by the estrogenic action of tamoxifen and not by endometrial proliferation.

In conclusion, an abnormally low uterine and endometrial vascular impedance in women receiving tamoxifen is not always pathological. Nevertheless, further studies in large series of patients are needed to clarify the clinical value of color Doppler flow in the differential diagnosis of endometrial neoplasia in these patients.

References

1. Sunderland, M. C. and Osborne, C. K. (1991). Tamoxifen in premenopausal patients with metastatic breast cancer: a review. *J. Clin. Oncol.*, **9**, 1283–97

2. Jordan, V. C. (1994). Molecular mechanisms of antiestrogen action in breast cancer. *Breast Cancer Res. Treat.*, **31**, 41–52

3. Friedl, A. and Jordan, V. C. (1994). What do we know and what don't we know about tamoxifen in human uterus? *Breast Cancer Res. Treat.*, **31**, 27–39

4. Quinn, M. and Allen, E. (1995). Changes in incidence of and mortality from breast cancer in England and Wales since introduction of screening. *Br. Med. J.*, **311**, 1391–5

5. Kedar, R. P., Bourne, T. H., Powles, T. J., Collins, W. P., Ashley, S. E., Cosgrove, D. O. and Campbell, S. (1994). Effects of tamoxifen on uterus and ovaries of postmenopausal women in a randomised breast cancer prevention trial. *Lancet*, **343**, 1318–21

6. Powles, T. J., Jones, A. L., Ashley, S. E., O'Brien, M. E. R., Tidy, V. A., Treleavan, J., Cosgrove, D. O., Sacks, N., Baum, M., McKinna, J. A. and Davey, J. B. (1994). The Royal Marsden Hospital pilot tamoxifen chemoprevention trial. *Breast Cancer Res. Treat.*, **31**, 73–82

7. Götzinger, P., Gnant, M., Hochstöger, E. and Jakesz, R. (1993). The potential impact of tamoxifen in breast cancer prevention. *Onkologie*, **16**, 297–303

8. Neven, P., Shepherd, J. H. and Lowe, D. G. (1993). Tamoxifen and the gynaecologist. *Br. J. Obstet. Gynaecol.*, **100**, 893–7

9. Marshal, E. (1995). Reanalysis confirms results of tained study. *Science*, **270**, 1562

10. Osborne, C. K. and Fuqua, S. A. W. (1994). Mechanism of tamoxifen resistance. *Breast Cancer Res. Treat.*, **32**, 49–55

11. Powles, T. J. and Hickish, T. (1995). Tamoxifen therapy and carcinogenic risk. *J. Natl. Cancer Inst.*, **87**, 1343–5

12. Gottardis, M. M., Robinson, S. P., Satyaswaroop, P. G. and Jordan, V. C. (1988). Contrasting actions of tamoxifen on endometrial and breast tumor in the athymic mouse. *Cancer Res.*, **48**, 812–15

13. Jordan, C. V. (1995). Tamoxifen and tumorigenicity: a predictable concern. *J. Natl. Cancer Inst.*, **87**, 623–6

14. Rutqvist, L. E., Johansson, H., Signomklao, T., Johansson, U., Fornander, T. and Wilking, N. (1995). Adjuvant tamoxifen therapy for early stage breast cancer and secondary primary malignancies. *J. Natl. Cancer Inst.*, **87**, 645–51

15. Jordan, V. C. (1993). How safe is tamoxifen. *Br. Med. J.*, **307**, 1371–2

16. Breast Cancer Trials Committee, Scottish Cancer Trials Office (MCR), Edinburgh (1987). Adjuvant tamoxifen in the management of operable breast cancer: The Scottish Trial. *Lancet*, **2**, 171–5

17. Malfetano, J. H. (1990). Tamoxifen-associated endometrial carcinoma in postmenopausal breast cancer patients. *Gynecol. Oncol.*, **39**, 82–3

18. Fonander, T., Cedermark, B., Mattsson, A., Skoog, L., Theve, T., Askergren, J., Rutqvist, L. E., Glas, U., Silfversward, C., Wilking, N. and Hjalmar, M. L. (1989). Adjuvant tamoxifen in early breast cancer: occurrence of new primary cancers. *Lancet*, **1**, 117–19

19. Wolf, D. M. and Jordan, V. C. (1992). Gynecologic complications associated with long-term adjuvant tamoxifen therapy for breast cancer. *Gynecol. Oncol.*, **45**, 118–28

20. Cohen, I., Rosen, J. D., Shapira, J., Cordoba, M., Gilboa, S., Altaras, M. M., Yigael, D. and Beyeth, Y. (1993). Endometrial changes in postmenopausal women treated with tamoxifen for breast cancer. *Br. J. Obstet. Gynaecol.*, **100**, 567–70

21. Ugwumadu, A. (1993). Endometrial changes and lesions in postmenopausal women treated with tamoxifen. *Br. J. Obstet. Gynaecol.*, **100**, 704–5

22. Magriples, U., Naftolin, F., Schwartz, P. E. and Carcangiu, M. L. (1993). High-grade endometrial carcinoma in tamoxifen-treated breast cancer patients. *J. Clin. Oncol.*, **11**, 485–90

23. Deprest, J., Neven, P. and Ide, P. (1992). An unusual type of endometrial cancer, related to tamoxifen? *Eur. J. Obstet. Gynecol. Reprod. Biol.*, **46**, 147–50

24. Seoud, M., Johnson, J. and Weed, J. C. (1993). Gynecologic tumors in tamoxifen-treated women with breast cancer. *Obstet. Gynecol.*, **82**, 165–9

25. Uziely, B., Lewin, A., Brufman, G., Dorembus, D. and Mor-Yosef, S. (1993). The effect of tamoxifen on the endometrium. *Breast Cancer Res. Treat.*, **26**, 101–5

26. Lahti, E., Blanco, G., Kauppila, A., Apaja-Sarkkinen, M., Taskinen, P. J. and Laatikainen, T. (1993). Endometrial changes in postmenopausal breast cancer patients receiving tamoxifen. *Obstet. Gynecol.*, **81**, 660–4

27. Neven, P. (1993). Tamoxifen and endometrial lesions. *Lancet*, **342**, 452

28. Ciatto, S., Cecchini, S., Bonardi, R. and Grazzini, G. (1994). Ultrasonography surveillance of endometrium in breast cancer patients on adjuvant tamoxifen. *Lancet*, **344**, 60

29. Cohen, I., Rosen, J. D., Shapira, J., Cordoba, M., Gilboa, S., Altaras, M. M., Dror, Y., and Beyeth, Y. (1994). Endometrial changes with tamoxifen: comparison between tamoxifen-treated and nontreated asymptomatic, postmenopausal breast cancer patients. *Gynecol. Oncol.*, **52**, 185–90

30. Van Leeuwen, F. E., Benraadt, J., Coebrgh, J. W. W., Kiemeney, L. A. L. M., Gimbrère, C. H. F., Otter, R., Schouten, L. J., Damhuis, R. A. M., Bontenbal, M., Diepenhorst, F. W., van den Belt-Dusebout, A. W. and van Tinteren, H. (1994). Risk of endometrial cancer after

tamoxifen treatment of breast cancer. *Lancet*, **343**, 448–52

31. Cohen, I., Tepper, R., Rosen, J. D., Shapira, J., Cordoba, M., Dror, Y., Altaras, M. M. and Beyeth, Y. (1994). Continuous tamoxifen treatment in asymptomatic, postmenopausal breast cancer patients does not cause aggravation of endometrial pathologies. *Gynecol. Oncol.*, **55**, 138–43

32. Cook, L. S., Weiss, N. S., Schwartz, S. M., White, E., McKnight, B., Moore, D. E. and Daling, J. R. (1995). Population-based study of tamoxifen therapy and subsequent ovarian, endometrial, and breast cancers. *J. Natl. Cancer Inst.*, **87**, 1359–64

33. Robinson, D. C., Bloss, J. D. and Schiano, M. A. (1995). A retrospective study of tamoxifen and endometrial cancer in breast cancer patients. *Gynecol. Oncol.*, **59**, 186–90

34. Le Bouedec, G., Pingeon, J. M. Fondrinier, E., Kauffmann, P. and Dauplat, J. (1995). Surveillance gynécologique des traitements du cancer du sein par le tamoxifène. *Rev. Fr. Gynécol. Obstét.*, **90**, 7–9

35. Neven, P., Aleem, F. A. and Predanic, M. (1995). Endometrial changes in patients on tamoxifen. *Lancet*, **346**, 1292–3

36. Fabian, C. J. (1995). Long-term tamoxifen treatment for breast cancers. *J. Natl. Cancer Inst.*, **87**, 1176–7

37. Lien, E. A., Anker, G. and Ueland, P. M. (1995). Pharmacokinetics of tamoxifen in premenopausal and postmenopausal women with breast cancer. *J. Steroid Biochem. Molec. Biol.*, **55**, 229–31

38. Fisher, B., Costantino, J. P., Redmond, C. K., Fisher, E. R., Wicherham, L. and Cronin, W. M. (1994). Endometrial cancer in tamoxifen treated breast cancer patients: findings from the National Adjuvant Breast and Bowel Project (NSABP-14). *J. Natl. Cancer Inst.*, **86**, 527–80

39. Bourne, T. H. (1995). Evaluating the endometrium of postmenopausal women with transvaginal ultrasonography. *Ultrasound Obstet. Gynecol.*, **6**, 75–80

40. Fleischer, A. C., Gordon, A. N., Entman, S. S. and Kepple, M. (1990). Transvaginal scanning of the endometrium. *J. Clin. Ultrasound*, **18**, 337–49

41. Goldstein, S. R., Nachtingal, M., Snyder, J. R. and Nachtingal, L. (1990). Endometrial assessment by vaginal ultrasonography before endometrial sampling in patients with postmenopausal bleeding. *Am. J. Obstet. Gynecol.*, **163**, 119–23

42. Wikland, M., Grandberg, S. and Karlsson, B. (1992). Assessment of the endometrium in the postmenopausal woman by vaginal sonography. *Ultrasound Q.*, **10**, 15–27

43. Osmers, R. (1992). Transvaginal sonography in the endometrial cancer. *Ultrasound Obstet. Gynecol.*, **2**, 2–3

44. Dørum, A., Kristensen, G. B., Langebrekke Sørness, T. and Skaar, O. (1993). Evaluation of endometrial thickness measured by endovaginal ultrasound in women with postmenopausal bleeding. *Acta Obstet. Gynecol. Scand.*, **72**, 116–19

45. Sheth, S., Hamper, U. M. and Kurman, R. J. (1993). Thickened endometrium in the postmenopausal woman: sonographic–pathologic correlation. *Radiology*, **187**, 135–9

46. Kurjak, A., Jurkovic, D., Alfirevic, Z. and Zalud, I. (1990). Transvaginal color Doppler imaging. *J. Clin. Ultrasound*, **18**, 227–34

47. Bourne, T. H., Campbell, S., Steer, C. V., Royston, P., Whitehead, M. I. and Collins, W. P. (1991). Detection of endometrial cancer by transvaginal ultrasound with color flow imaging and blood flow analysis: a preliminary report. *Gynecol. Oncol.*, **40**, 253–9

48. Kurjak, A., Shalan, H., Sosic, A., Benic, S., Zudenigo, D., Kupesic, S. and Predanic, M. (1993). Endometrial carcinoma in postmenopausal women: evaluation by transvaginal color Doppler ultrasonography. *Am. J. Obstet. Gynecol.*, **169**, 1597–603

49. Kupesic-Urek, S., Shalan, H. and Kurjak, A. (1993). Early detection of endometrial cancer by transvaginal color Doppler. *Eur. J. Obstet. Gynecol. Reprod. Biol.*, **49**, 46–9

50. Carter, J., Saltzman, A., Hartenbach, E., Fowler, J., Carson, L. and Twiggs, L. B. (1994). Flow characteristics in benign and malignant tumors using transvaginal color flow Doppler. *Obstet. Gynecol.*, **83**, 125–30

51. Loeffer, F. D. (1989). Hysteroscopy with selective endometrial sampling compared with D&C for abnormal uterine bleeding: the value of negative hysteroscopic view. *Obstet. Gynecol.*, **73**, 16–20

52. Valle, R. F. (1991). Hysteroscopy. *Curr. Opinion Obstet. Gynecol.*, **3**, 422–6

53. Gimpelson, R. J. (1992). Office hysteroscopy. *Clin. Obstet. Gynecol.*, **35**, 270–81

54. Mencaglia, L. (1995). Hysteroscopy and adenocarcinoma. *Obstet. Gynecol. Clin. North Am.*, **22**, 573–9

55. De Muylder, X., Neven, P., De Somer, M., Van Belle, Y., Vanderick, G., and De Muylder, E. (1991). Endometrial lesions in patients undergoing tamoxifen therapy. *Int. J. Gynecol. Obstet.*, **36**, 127–30

56. Neven, P., De Muylder, X., Van Belle, Y., Vanderick, G. and De Muylder, E. (1990). Hysteroscopic follow-up during tamoxifen treatment. *Eur. J. Obstet. Gynecol. Reprod. Biol.*, **35**, 235–8

57. Hulka, C. A. and Hall, D. A. (1993). Endometrial abnormalities associated with tamoxifen therapy for breast cancer: sonographic and pathologic correlation. *Am. J. Roentgenol.*, **160**, 809–12

58. Corley, D., Rowe, J., Curtis, M. T., Hogan, W. M., Noumoff, J. S. and Livolsi, V. A. (1992). Postmenopausal bleeding from unusual endometrial polyps in women on chronic tamoxifen therapy. *Obstet. Gynecol.*, **79**, 111–16

59. Goldstein, S. R. (1994). Unusual ultrasonographic appearance of the uterus in patients receiving tamoxifen. *Am. J. Obstet. Gynecol.*, **170**, 447–51

60. Perrot, N., Guyot, B., Antoine, M. and Uzan, S. (1994). The effects of tamoxifen on the endometrium. *Ultrasound Obstet. Gynecol.*, **4**, 83–4

61. Nuovo, M. A., Nuovo, G. J., McCaffrey, R. M., Levine, R. U., Barron, B. and Winkler, B. (1989). Endometrial polyps in postmenopausal patients receiving tamoxifen. *Int. J. Gynecol. Pathol.*, **8**, 125–31

62. Exacoustòs, C., Zupi, E., Cangi, B., Chiaretti, M., Arduini, D. and Romanini, C. (1995). Endometrial evaluation in postmenopausal breast cancer patients receiving tamoxifen: an ultrasound, color flow Doppler, hysteroscopic and histological study. *Ultrasound Obstet. Gynecol.*, **6**, 435–42

63. Tepper, R., Cohen, I., Altaras, M., Shapira, J., Cordoba, M., Dror, Y. and Beyth, Y. (1995). Doppler flow evaluation of pathologic endometrial conditions in postmenopausal breast cancer patients treated with tamoxifen. *J. Clin. Ultrasound.*, **13**, 635–40

64. Mazur, M. T. and Kurman, R. J. (1995). *Diagnosis of Endometrial Biopsies and Curettings*, pp. 102–3, 120–3, 146–59. (Berlin: Springer Verlag)

65. Achiron, R., Lipitz, S., Sivan, E., Goldenberg, M., Horovitz, A., Frenkel, Y. and Mashiach, S. (1995). Changes mimicking endometrial neoplasia in postmenopausal, tamoxifen-treated women with breast cancer: a transvaginal Doppler study. *Ultrasound Obstet. Gynecol.*, **6**, 116–20

66. Achiron, R., Grisaru, D., Golan-Porat, N. and Lipitz, S. (1996). Tamoxifen and the uterus: an old drug tested by new modalities. *Ultrasound Obstet. Gynecol.*, **7**, 374–8

67. Uzan, S., Perrot, N. and Uzan, M. (1992). Tamoxifen: vaginosonography and color Doppler assessment of the uterus. *Ultrasound Obstet. Gynecol.*, **3**, 306

68. Bourne, T., Hillard, T. C., Whitehead, M. I., Crook, D. and Campbell, S. (1990). Oestrogens, arterial status, and postmenopausal women. *Lancet*, **335**, 1470–1

69. Pirhonen, J. P., Vuento, M. H., Måkinen, J. I. and Salmi, T. A. (1993). Long-term effects of hormone replacement therapy on the uterus and on uterine circulation. *Am. J. Obstet. Gynecol.*, **168**, 620–3

70. Achiron, R., Lipitz, S., Frenkel, Y. and Mashiach, S. (1995). Endometrial blood flow response to estrogen replacement therapy and tamoxifen in asymptomatic, postmenopausal women: a transvaginal Doppler study. *Ultrasound Obstet. Gynecol.*, **5**, 411–14

71. Weiner, Z., Beck, D., Rottem, S., Brandes, J. M. and Thaler, I. (1993). Uterine artery flow velocity waveforms and color flow imaging in women with perimenopausal and postmenopausal bleeding. Correlation to endometrial histopathology. *Acta Obstet. Gynecol. Scand.*, **72**, 162–6

72. Carter, J. R., Lau, M., Saltzman, A. K., Hartenbach, E. M., Chen, M. D., Johnson, P. R., Fowler, J. M., Carlson, J. W., Carson, L. F. and Twiggs, L. B. (1994). Gray scale and color flow Doppler characterization of uterine tumors. *J. Clin. Ultrasound*, **13**, 835–40

73. Exacoustòs, C., Chiaretti, M., Cangi, B., Zupi, E., Arduini, D. and Romanini, C. (1994). Screening for endometrial cancer: transvaginal color Doppler sonographic findings in postmenopausal patients. *Ultrasound Obstet. Gynecol.*, **4**, suppl.1, 132

Transvaginal sonography and endometrial biopsy in peri- and postmenopausal women with vaginal bleeding

6

T. J. Dubinsky

INTRODUCTION

Peri- and postmenopausal vaginal bleeding (PMB) is one of the most frequent reasons for women to seek medical attention, and it accounts for approximately 5% of all gynecological visits in the United States. As our population ages and as life expectancy continues to grow, the number of women over age 55 is expected to grow from 30 million to 45 million by the year 2020[1]. Women placed on hormone replacement therapy for the treatment of PMB, or a tamoxifen regimen for breast carcinoma have an increased risk of endometrial carcinoma that must be evaluated annually. All of these factors are placing greater demand on our health-care system to care for PMB patients at a time when health care resources are becoming more limited.

Historically, women presenting with PMB underwent hysterectomies, and, in part due to PMB, hysterectomy became the most commonly performed surgical procedure in the United States. However, the morbidity and cost associated with a major surgical procedure make hysterectomy an undesirable choice for treating PMB in most cases. The ability to utilize ultrasound to diagnose the various etiologies of PMB, the development of estrogen replacement therapy, and the utilization of hysteroscopy have significantly reduced the demand for hysterectomy, and subsequently the cost of PMB-related health care. The evaluation of women with PMB will require increasingly more efficient diagnostic and therapeutic methods to achieve the necessary cost effectiveness while maintaining high quality as the standard of care.

ETIOLOGY OF PERI- AND POSTMENOPAUSAL VAGINAL BLEEDING

Atrophic endometritis is responsible for approximately 30% of PMB[2]. In 1966, it was proposed that many of the symptoms in aging women could be attributed to estrogen deficiency, including PMB[3]. Subsequently it was discovered that the use of estrogen, particularly unopposed estrogen (without progesterone) increased a woman's risk for endometrial carcinoma[4]. Therefore, in recent years, exogenous estrogens with varying combinations of progesterone have been used to treat women with PMB and it is estimated 20–30% of all women with PMB are being treated in this manner[1]. Due to the increased risk of endometrial carcinoma associated with the use of the hormone therapy, many gynecologists now recommend yearly endometrial biopsies in these women. Evidence is beginning to accumulate that indicates that transvaginal sonography (TVS) is a more effective means for screening for carcinoma than endometrial biopsy.

Of all PMB, true endometrial or endoluminal etiologies account for only 30–40% of the cases including endometrial hyperplasia (10%),

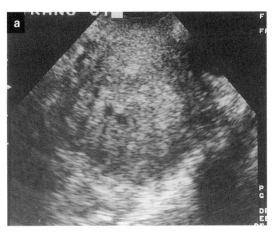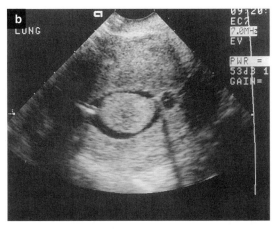

Figure 1 (a) A pre-saline infusion image demonstrating a 2.1 cm thick endometrium in a postmenopausal woman with 6 months of irregular bleeding and two prior negative EMB. (b) The post-saline image demonstrates that the entire endometrial canal is occupied by a large echogenic mass proved to be an adenomatous polyp at hysteroscopic removal

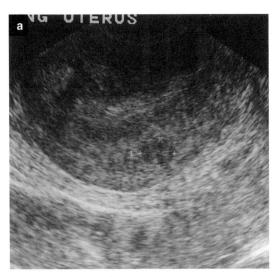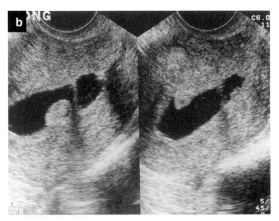

Figure 2 (a) A woman with 3 months of bleeding and a prior positive EMB for a polyp. The pre-saline infusion image demonstrates a 1.2 cm thick endometrium. (b) The post-saline image demonstrates two different polyps. Twenty five per cent of the hysterosonograms we have performed have demonstrated more than one lesion. This patient had both polyps removed hysteroscopically and her bleeding stopped

endometrial polyps (10%) (Figures 1–3), endoluminal fibromyomata (10%) (Figure 4) and uterine malignancies (10%)[5] (Figure 5). Most of the cancers responsible for PMB are endometrial in origin, accounting for 5–8% of all causes of PMB. Endometrial carcinoma is, therefore, the most important etiology of PMB that must be excluded, and, if detected early, endometrial carcinoma is the most treatable of all the female genital carcinomas, with a survival rate of greater than 80% for stage I disease. Since PMB can be secondary to either benign or malignant conditions, it has become the standard of care to exclude the possibility of malignancy histologically prior to investigating other etiologies for PMB. Hence, some form of endometrial biopsy, whether dilatation and curettage (D & C), aspiration endometrial biopsy, or

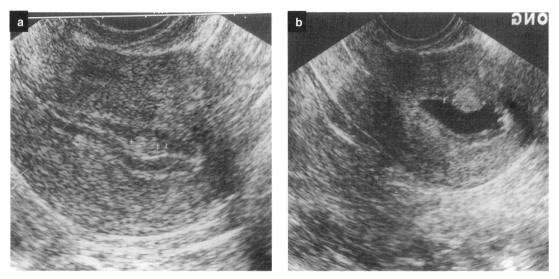

Figure 3 (a) A mid-sagittal image demonstrating a focal echogenic mass in the posterior endometrial wall in an asymptomatic woman. (b) The post-saline image confirms the presence of a small polyp. It is not entirely clear at this time if these should be removed, or followed with TVS

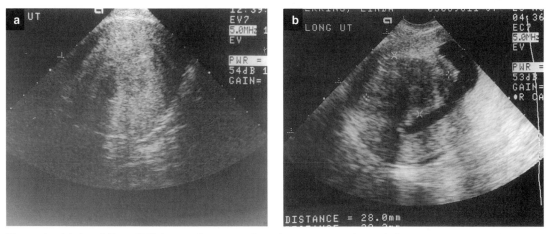

Figure 4 (a) An oblique TVS image demonstrating what appears to be an inhomogeneous mass displacing the endometrium anteriorly. This was felt to be a polyp or carcinoma. This patient was bleeding, and had had a negative EMB and D & C. (b) The post-saline infusion image shows that this is in fact a submucosal fibroid located in the anterior wall. Women such as this may not need any biopsy procedure, and instead can probably undergo myotomy or hysterectomy

hysteroscopically guided D & C is nearly always performed as part of the evaluation of PMB. As the ultrasound diagnosis of all of these conditions continues to improve, and outperform biopsy techniques, questions arise concerning the validity of always performing a biopsy or D & C as the initial examination rather than transvaginal sonography.

DILATATION AND CURETTAGE

In the past, endometrial biopsies were performed primarily by D & C, where the cervix is dilated under anesthesia, and the endometrium is scraped with a spoon-like probe[6]. Initial reports were optimistic about the accuracy of D & C for the diagnosis of endometrial

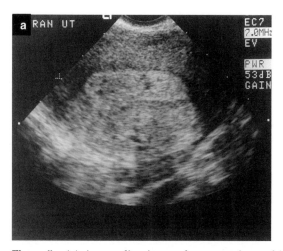 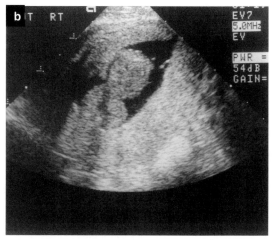

Figure 5 (a) A pre-saline image demonstrating a thickened endometrium with several small cystic spaces within it. This patient had not had a biopsy. (b) The post-saline image shows a dumb-bell-shaped lesion within the endometrial canal that was felt to represent a polyp but was interpreted as carcinoma at pathology

carcinomas with false-negative rates of 2–6%[7,8]. A therapeutic effect of D & C for PMB was also reported, and then discounted[9]. Recent investigations have raised doubt with regard to the utility of D & C for demonstrating many endoluminal lesions including a recent study by Carlsson and co-workers[10] who compared the combination of transvaginal ultrasound and hysteroscopy to D & C. They found that, in 11 of 12 patients, when the ultrasound was normal, the histology obtained at hysteroscopy was also normal (one small polyp was found at hysteroscopy that was not seen with ultrasound). In 35 of 39 patients with a thickened endometrium as seen with ultrasound, histological specimens were also abnormal (with four false-positive). In nine cases, polyps were found on both transvaginal sonography and hysteroscopy following a negative D & C. Gimpleson and Rappold studied 276 patients and found that in 44 patients hysteroscopy was more accurate than D & C versus nine cases when D & C was more accurate[11]. It has been estimated that D & C samples only 60% of the endometrial surface[12,13], so it is apparent that there is significant potential to miss endometrial pathology, particularly pedunculated lesions such as polyps and submucosal fibroids that can move away from instruments and which are subsequently difficult to diagnose by D & C[10]. It has generally been assumed that

D & C is more effective for diffuse rather than focal endometrial disorders such as hyperplasia and carcinoma, yet many patients with PMB whose initial endometrial biopsy or D & C reveals benign or insufficient tissue may eventually be diagnosed with endometrial cancer or complex endometrial hyperplasia[14].

ENDOMETRIAL ASPIRATION BIOPSY

The technique of aspiration endometrial biopsy (EMB) was subsequently developed with the advantage that it did not require anesthesia, was cheaper, and could be performed more easily in the outpatient setting than D & C. The technique involves placing a catheter with multiple side holes attached to a vacu-lok syringe through the cervix into the uterus. The syringe is then aspirated while being moved back and forth. Initial results indicated that EMB can diagnose 80–85% of endometrial cancers, but several recent investigations have indicated a lower sensitivity[15]. Endometrial biopsies miss endometrial lesions since they are performed 'blindly', and sample only a small portion of the total endometrial surface. In addition, as with D & C, pedunculated lesions can move away from the biopsy instrument, and incipient polyps may not be identified if the basal layer of the endometrium is not included in the specimen[16].

TRANSVAGINAL SONOGRAPHY

Paralleling the advances in endometrial biopsy techniques, developments in transvaginal ultrasound have made it widely accepted as the modality of choice for imaging the uterus and the endometrium. Numerous recent publications[5,17,18] have indicated that transvaginal ultrasonography is an effective procedure with which to exclude endometrial and intrauterine abnormalities, and its use is advocated as a routine first-step procedure in patients with abnormal uterine bleeding. Recent investigators have shown that when the endometrium is less than 4 mm thick, biopsy specimens return as normal, or as insufficient tissue, with a specificity of 95% for endometrial carcinoma[19]. Thickening of the endometrium greater than 5 mm has been shown to be a sensitive finding for detecting endometrial pathology, and the incidence of endometrial carcinoma is higher in women in whom the endometrium is thicker than 5 mm[20,21] with a greater than 90% sensitivity[20,21]. Hence, several publications have shown that the sensitivity of TVS is greater than the most optimistic reports regarding EMB and D & C.

Unfortunately, hyperplasia, polyps, and carcinoma all present as endometrial thickening. Additional ultrasound imaging observations such as the presence of cysts and degree of endometrial inhomogeneity[22,23] and color flow/duplex imaging[24,25] have been utilized to improve this relative lack of specificity. TVS can be used accurately, as a first step screening procedure to determine which patients should undergo further investigation.

TRANSVAGINAL SONOGRAPHY VERSUS ENDOMETRIAL ASPIRATION BIOPSY

Despite the large number of recent publications advocating ultrasound[26], EMB is still currently considered by most gynecologists to be the standard of care as the initial diagnostic procedure of choice in the evaluation of PMB. Shipley and co-workers[27] compared EMB with transvaginal ultrasound in 50 asymptomatic women; seven of nine women had abnormal endometrial thickening on TVS following a negative EMB, one woman had an abnormal TVS and EMB, and another had a normal ultrasound with a positive EMB. All nine women subsequently had histologic confirmation of endometrial pathology, either by D & C or by hysteroscopy. It has generally been assumed that the sensitivity of EMB was comparable to that of D & C, yet it is becoming increasingly clear that this is not the case. TVS appears to have far better sensitivity than EMB although as a result of this improved sensitivity more false-positive diagnoses occur.

Recently, several investigators including ourselves[28,29] have reported the utility of hysterosonography, a technique whereby the endometrial canal is filled with sterile saline under ultrasound visualization, for improving the specificity of endometrial ultrasound imaging, and for helping to distinguish between the varying etiologies for PMB. Several authors have demonstrated that filling the endometrial cavity with fluids allows improved detection and delineation of small endoluminal masses such as polyps and cancers that may otherwise escape detection with TVS alone. Hysterosonography can show the size, location and attachment of endometrial lesions, and it can exclude masses in women who appear to have thickened endometria on transvaginal ultrasound.

HYSTEROSONOGRAPHY VERSUS ENDOMETRIAL ASPIRATION BIOPSY

By utilizing transvaginal hysterosonography (TVHS) we later discovered that in 41 cases, endometrial pathology was missed by biopsy including polyps, carcinomas (Figure 5), and hyperplasia in women with PMB[30]. All of these lesions were detected on transvaginal sonography as thickening of the endometrium, and these lesions were remarkably well seen on hysterosonography. In our original series, 29 patients of 48 with endometrial thickening on transvaginal sonography had no abnormality identified on hysterosonography. As our experience grew, our false-positive examinations diminished so that in our second series, only seven of an additional 33 patients with endometrial thickening had negative hysterosonography. We also found that using a cut-off of 7 mm instead of 5 mm for endometrial thickness eliminated 83 of the false-positive TVS examinations. In our experience the number of false-positive TVS examinations is reduced by saline infusion thus improving the specificity of transvaginal ultrasound. Our study also raised suspicion about the utility of EMB versus TVS in the evaluation of PMB, but a significant selection bias was present in this study since patients were selected on the basis of prior negative EMB.

Subsequently the database was expanded by reviewing all of the pathology results for all of the EMBs performed during the last 2 years on women older than 45 years. The sensitivity of biopsy for the detection of all endometrial pathology was only 30%, for carcinoma 50%, and for hyperplasia 70%. As of this time, biopsy has missed seven carcinomas which were demonstrated with hysterosonography (Figure 6). In 60% of cases, biopsies were performed on women who would not have needed one given ultrasound findings indicative of submucosal fibroids or endometrial atrophy. We have also found three uterine sarcomas in women with negative biopsies. It is women with fibroids and atrophy that account for the majority of PMB, and TVS is clearly a more effective means for establishing these diagnoses than biopsy.

HYSTEROSCOPY

Ultimately, the diagnosis of proven endometrial lesions as demonstrated by TVS requires a biopsy specimen for a histologic evaluation, and hysteroscopy has emerged as the most promising technique for obtaining such specimens. Hysteroscopy allows a directed biopsy of visualized lesions, and it can be performed in an outpatient setting. While of great utility, it is of considerably greater expense than is ultrasound, and it has greater risks, including uterine perforation, than does hysterosonography. It has not been established whether TVHS needs to be performed prior to hysteroscopy in every case, or if it should be reserved for those cases when hysteroscopy fails to resolve PMB, but the presence of a 10–20% false-positive rate with TVS suggests that hysterosonography should be performed prior to more invasive procedures (Figure 7). Given that nearly 60% of patients will have ultrasound findings that obviate the need for biopsy, it will probably not be feasible to use hysteroscopy as a screening examination in women with PMB.

TRANSVAGINAL SONOGRAPHY VERSUS HYSTEROSCOPY

In our most recent study, 25% of our patients had multiple lesions demonstrated with hystero-

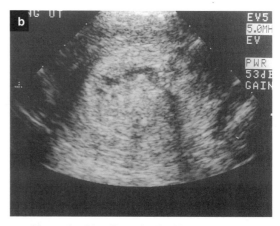

Figure 6 (a) A pre-saline image in a woman with 2 years of irregular bleeding who had had an EMB and a D & C interpreted as hyperplasia. (b) The saline infusion image shows an irregular polypoid mass that was a carcinoma at pathology. Several areas of endometrial thickening are evident and were hyperplasia. It is apparent from this image how a reading of hyperplasia occurred in the presence of a carcinoma

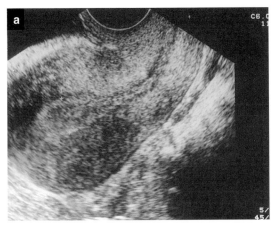 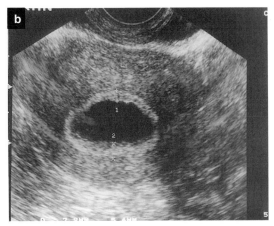

Figure 7 (a) A pre-saline image showing 1.2 cm of inhomogeneous endometrial thickening. The patient had had 5 months of bleeding, and a negative EMB. (b) No lesion is identified within the lumen. We have seen endometrial thickening on TVS without a true lesion on saline infusion in 10% of our cases (depending on what thickness is used as a cut-off for performing saline infusion). Hence, we believe that hysterosonography improves the specificity of TVS as well as aiding in the differentiation of the numerous etiologies of endometrial thickening which is a non-specific finding

sonography. It is not clear whether all of them would have been seen with hysteroscopy. Even if EMB had been positive in these cases, the multiple pathologic lesions may not have been detected, and it is not clear whether PMB would resolve following hysteroscopic removal of a single polyp in these cases. Many patients with endometrial thickening will prove to have submucosal fibroids, and these patients will probably not need hysteroscopy to resect these fibroids. In some patients, particularly those with lesions suspicious for carcinoma, perhaps hysterectomy would be more appropriate than hysteroscopy. Prospective blinded comparisons between hysteroscopy and hysterosonography will be necessary to completely establish the role of each in the evaluation of PMB.

CONCLUSION

The evaluation of endometrial disorders in all women including those with PMB continues to evolve, and it appears that TVS, particularly in combination with TVHS, has an essential role in screening for those patients who will need further diagnostic evaluation, and in determining which of several procedure options will benefit the patient most. With an enlarging population of postmenopausal women, and with women being treated with hormone replacement and tamoxifen therapy, the number of examinations performed specifically to evaluate endometrial disorders will also increase. The application of TVS to premenopausal women with dysfunctional uterine bleeding to differentiate women with endoluminal lesions from those with primary amenorrhea will probably also increase. The role of TVS/TVHS with regard to hysteroscopy still needs to be studied, although it appears obvious that TVS will be more cost effective for screening of PMB. In summary, TVS has emerged as the least invasive, most sensitive means to assess the endometrium, particularly in combination with hysterosonography, and a large body of evidence exists indicating that TVS should be performed prior to any type of biopsy procedure, particularly in women with PMB.

References

1. Lobo, R. A. (1995). Benefits and risk of estrogen replacement therapy. *Am. J. Obstet. Gynecol.*, **173**, 982–9

2. Kazadi-Buanga, J. and Jurado-Chacon, M. (1994). Etiologic study of 275 cases of endo-uterine hemorrhage by uterine curettage. *Rev. Fr. Gynecol. Obstet.*, **89**, 129

3. Wilson, R. A. (1966). *Feminine Forever.* (New York: Evans)

4. World Health Organization Scientific Group (1981). *Research on the Menopause*, pp. 53–68. (Geneva: World Health Organization)

5. Granberg, S., Wikland, K., Darlsson, B. *et al.* (1991). Endometrial thickness as measured by endovaginal ultrasonography for identifying endometrial abnormality. *Am. J. Obstet. Gynecol.*, **164**, 47

6. Stowall, T. G., Solomon, S. K. and Ling, F. W. (1989). Endometrial sampling prior to hyster-ectomy. *Obstet. Gynecol.*, **73**, 405

7. Bistoletti, P., Hjerpe, A. and Mollerstrom, G. (1988). Cytological diagnosis of endometrial cancer and preinvasive endometrial lesions. *Acta Obstet. Gynecol. Scand.*, **67**, 342

8. McKenzie, I. Z. and Bibby, J. G. (1978). Critical assessment of dilatations and curettage in 1029 women. *Lancet*, **332**, 566

9. Taylor, P. J. and Graham, G. (1982). Is diagnostic curettage harmful to women with unexplained infertility? *Br. J. Obstet. Gynaecol.*, **89**, 296–8

10. Carlsson, B., Granberg, S., Hellberg, P. and Wikland, M. (1994). Comparative study of trans-vaginal sonography and hysteroscopy for the detection of pathologic endometrial lesions in women with postmenopausal bleeding. *J. Ultra-sound Med.*, **13**, 757–62

11. Gimpleson, R. J. and Rappold, H. O. (1988). A comparative study between panoramic hystero-scopy with directed biopsies and dilatation and curettage. *Am. J. Obstet. Gynecol.*, **158**, 489

12. Word, B., Gravelee, L. C. and Wideman, G. L. (1958). The fallacy of simple uterine curettage. *Obstet. Gynecol.*, **12**, 642

13. Grimes, D. A. (1982). Diagnostic dilatation and curettage. A reappraisal. *Am. J. Obstet. Gynecol.*, **142**, 1

14. Feldman, S., Shapter, A., Welch, W. R. *et al.* (1994). Two year follow-up of 263 patients with post/perimenopausal vaginal bleeding and negative initial biopsy. *Gynecol. Oncol.*, **55**, 56

15. Larson, D. M., Krawisz, B. R., Johnson, K. K. *et al.* (1994). Comparison of the Z-sampler and Novak endometrial biopsy instruments for in-office diagnosis of endometrial cancer. *Gynecol. Oncol.*, **54**, 64

16. Kallenback Hellweg, G. C. (1987). The histo-pathology of the endometrium. 2. Functional endogenous (hormonal disturbance). Special forms of hyperplasia (focal hyperplasia, polyps, glandular and stromal hyperplasia). In *Histo-pathology of the Endometrium*, 4th edn. (Berlin: Springer-Verlag)

17. Fleischer, A. C., Mendelson, E. B., Bohm-Velez, M. *et al.* (1988). Transvaginal and transabdomi-nal sonography of the endometrium. *Semin. Ultrasound CT MR*, **98**, 81

18. Osmers, R., Volksen, M. and Schauer, A. L. (1990). Vaginosonography for early detection of endometrial carcinoma? *Lancet*, **335**, 1569

19. Karlsson, B., Granberg, S., Wikland, M., Ylostalo, P., Torvid, K., Marsal, K. and Valentin, L. (1995). Transvaginal ultrasonography of the endomet-rium in women with postmenopausal bleeding – a Nordic multicenter study. *Am. J. Obstet. Gynecol.*, **172**, 1488–94

20. Nasri, M. N., Shepherd, J. H., Setchell, M. E. *et al.* (1991). Sonographic depiction of post-menopausal endometrium with transabdominal and transvaginal scanning. *Ultrasound Obstet. Gynecol.*, **1**, 279

21. Nasri, M. N., Shepherd, J. H., Setchell, M. E. *et al.* (1991). The role of vaginal scanning in measurement of endometrial thickness in post-menopausal women. *Br. J. Obstet. Gynaecol.*, **98**, 470

22. Hulka, C. A., Hall, C. A., McCarthy, K. and Simeone, J. F. (1994). Endometrial polyps, hyperplasia, and carcinoma in postmenopausal women: differentiation with endovaginal sono-graphy. *Radiology*, **191**, 755–8

23. Sheth, S., Hamper, U. M. and Kurman, R. (1991). Thickened endometrium in the post-menopausal woman: sonographic-pathologic correlation. *Radiology*, **187**, 135

24. Bourne, T. H., Campbell, S., Whitehead, M. I. *et al.* (1990). Detection of endometrial cancer in postmenopausal women by transvaginal ultra-sonography and colour flow imaging. *Br. Med. J.*, **301**, 369

25. Kurjak, A., Predanic, M., Kupesic, S. *et al.* (1993). Transvaginal color and pulsed Doppler assess-ment of adnexal tumor vascularity. *Gynecol. Oncol.*, **50**, 3

26. Goldstein, S. R., Nachtigall, M., Snyder, J. R. *et al.* (1990). Endometrial assessment by vaginal ultra-sonography before endometrial sampling in

patients with postmenopausal bleeding. *Am. J. Obstet. Gynecol.,* **161**, 119

27. Shipley, C. F., Simmons, C. L. and Nelson, G. H. (1994). Comparison of transvaginal sonography with endometrial biopsy in asymptomatic post-menopausal women. *J. Ultrasound Med.,* **13**, 99–104

28. Parson, S. A. K. and Lense, J. J. (1993). Sono-hysterography for endometrial abnormalities: preliminary results. *J. Clin. Ultrasound,* **21**, 87

29. Dubinsky, T. J., Parvey, H. R., Gormaz, G. and Maklad, N. (1995). Transvaginal hysterosono-graphy in the evaluation of small endoluminal masses. *J. Ultrasound Med.,* **14**, 1

30. Dubinsky, T. J., Parvey, H. R., Gormaz, G., Curtis, M. and Maklad, N. (1995). Transvaginal hysterosonography: comparison with biopsy in the evaluation of postmenopausal bleeding. *J. Ultrasound Med.,* **14**, 887–93

Transvaginal sonography of endometrial cancer

7

A. C. Fleischer

INTRODUCTION

Endometrial cancer is the most common female genital cancer and will affect over 50 000 women this year, with over 3000 deaths in the United States. Although the 5-year survival of endometrial cancer patients has been improving, almost half of the women first diagnosed with the disease will have invasion into the myometrium, and 46% of these will have pelvic lymphadenopathy, with 29% having spread to the peri-aortic nodes[1].

Early and accurate diagnosis of endometrial carcinoma is of the utmost clinical importance in order to optimize long-term survival. Seventy-five to 80% of all cases occur after menopause, with the peak incidence occurring between 55 and 65 years of age. Only 67% of all histologically confirmed endometrial cancers can be diagnosed by exfoliative cytology[1]. Therefore, this procedure is not suitable for screening. The vast percentage of patients (85–95%) with endometrial cancer will present with bleeding as the first symptom. Hyperplasia is a known precursor to endometrial carcinoma. This condition can be suspected, based on transvaginal sonography, when the endometrium bilayer thickness measures over 5 mm and has an irregular texture[2].

Many studies have indicated that, when screening for endometrial cancer is combined with screening for ovarian cancer, approximately 1 in 2000 in the asymptomatic population and 1 in 250 in the symptomatic or high-risk population may have a sonographic abnormality requiring further evaluation[3–6]. Since transvaginal sonography is a good indicator of endometrial pathology in patients with bleeding, it can be used as a triage to identify women who may benefit from endometrial biopsy from those with a thin endometrium which suggests that bleeding is due to an atrophic endometritis[2].

SONOGRAPHIC DIFFERENTIAL DIAGNOSIS OF ENDOMETRIAL THICKENING

Endometrial thickening is defined based on the patient's menopausal status and whether or not she is taking hormone replacement medications. In the menstruating woman, endometrial thicknesses may extend up to 12–14 mm in the luteal phase, whereas in the postmenopausal patient, endometrial thicknesses of over 5 mm suggest an abnormality (Figures 1 and 2). Women on combined estrogen–progesterone hormone replacement may have endometria up to 8 mm[7–9]. One can use transvaginal sonography to monitor serially thickening of the endometrium in women on hormone replacement. Those on sequential estrogen–progesterone regimens may demonstrate up to 2 mm difference in thickness, depending on when they are studied[9].

Texture is also an important sonographic parameter in that polyps may appear as echogenic, polypoid lesions that may or may not have surrounding fluid to enhance their sonographic visualization. In some cases, sonohysterography may be useful to identify polypoid lesions. Cancer may be present in polyps, although it is rare.

Endometrial cancer typically produces endometrial thickness greater than 10 mm in the postmenopausal woman[10]. The endometrial

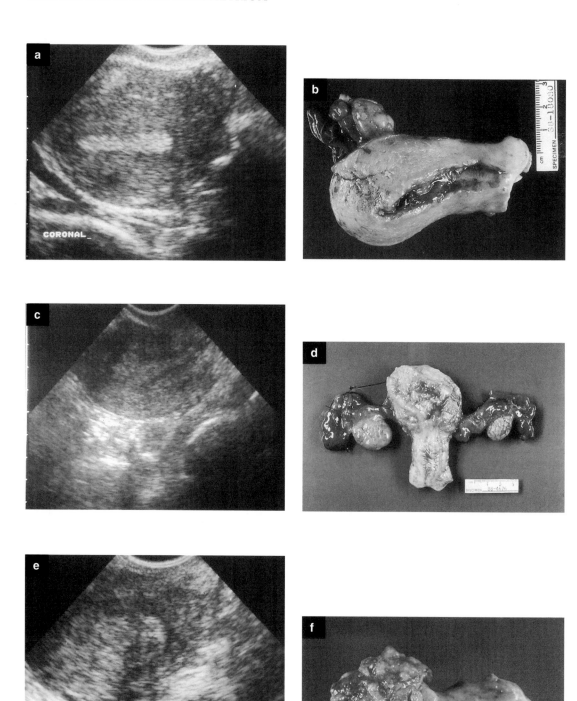

Figure 1 *See legend on next page*

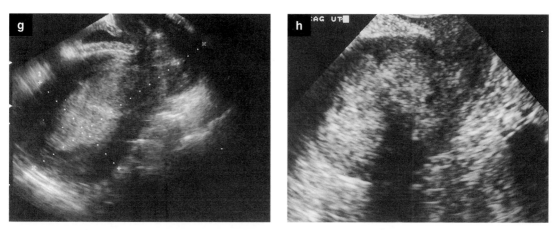

Figure 1 Transvaginal sonography of endometrial cancer with pathologic correlation. (a) Non-invasive: transvaginal sonography shows intact endometrial–myometrial interface; sectioned specimen (b) shows well-defined endometrial–myometrial interface and no gross myometrial invasion. (c) Moderately invasive: transvaginal sonography shows a disrupted endometrial–myometrial interface near the fundus; sectioned specimen (d) confirms myometrial invasion near the fundus. Extensively invasive: transvaginal sonography (e) shows extension of tumor to serosa near fundus; sectioned specimen (f) confirms extensive invasive tumor near fundus. (g) Transvaginal sonography of a polypoid cancer distending the endometrial lumen. On pathology, endometrial and squamous cell cancer were found. (h) Transvaginal sonography of an invasive endometrial cancer appearing as irregular and echogenic intraluminal and myometrial tissue

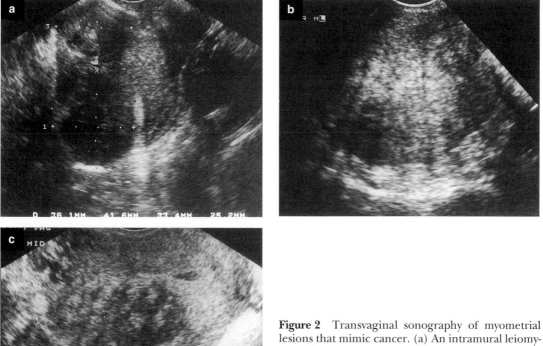

Figure 2 Transvaginal sonography of myometrial lesions that mimic cancer. (a) An intramural leiomyoma (between cursors) appearing as a hypoechoic myometrial mass that displaces the endometrium. (b) Diffuse adenomyomatosis appearing as diffusely echogenic and irregular myometrium. (c) A hypoechoic intramural leiomyoma that displaces the endometrium

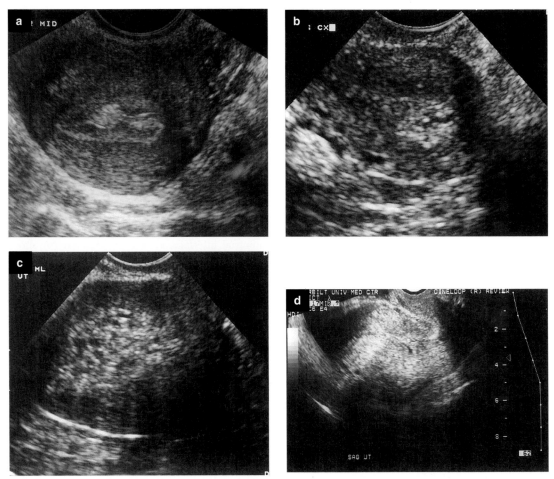

Figure 3 Discrepant transvaginal sonography and endometrial biopsy. (a) Sonography showing polyp effacing endometrial layers; endometrial biopsy was falsely negative. (b) Sonography showing a thickened and irregular endometrium containing cystic areas; biopsy revealed fragmented inactive endometrial glands negative for hyperplasia or cancer. (c) Thickened endometrium with punctate cystic areas in a patient on tamoxifen who had a negative biopsy. This was found to represent a large polyp containing numerous obstructed glands. (d) Polyp filling the endometrial lumen that contained a focus of clear cell carcinoma in a patient with a negative endometrial biopsy on tamoxifen

texture is typically irregular and may extend into the surrounding myometrial layers. Detailed evaluation of the myometrial layers with transvaginal sonography is important in that invasive disease has a worse prognosis and may require lymph node resection, whereas non-invasive disease is typically treated by simple hysterectomy. Radiation therapy may also be instituted if deep myometrial invasion is present. Invasion can be implied if there is a disruption in the endometrial–subendometrial myometrium layer. Rarely, other conditions, such as adenomyosis, may cause textural disturbance which

mimics that seen in invasive endometrial carcinoma[11].

Magnetic resonance provides a secondary means to assess myometrial involvement if transvaginal sonography is not definitive[12]. The ability to distinguish the inner myometrium is improved with the use of contrast enhancement.

MYOMETRIAL DISORDERS THAT MIMIC ENDOMETRIAL INVASION

Certain benign conditions produce irregularities in the myometrium that may mimic the sonographic appearance of invasive endometrial cancer. Foremost among these is adenomyosis, which represents endometrial tissue embedded within the myometrium. Adenomyosis may appear as an abnormally echogenic area within the myometrium on sonography[13,14]. With color Doppler sonography, a diffuse increase in vascularity may be seen in some cases, as opposed to the rim-like blood flow patterns in leiomyoma[15]. Rarely, adenomyosis may appear as an asymmetrical hypoechoic area[11].

Intramural leiomyoma are frequently causes of myometrial irregularity. In addition, their displacement of the endometrium can usually be outlined. Leiomyomas are usually hypoechoic when compared to the endometrium, and their whorled configuration can be ascertained (Figure 2c).

Tamoxifen may produce irregular cystic spaces within the inner myometrium[16]. Punctate hypoechoic areas may also be seen in polyps, representing obstructed glandular elements. There is an increased risk of endometrial cancer in these patients[17,18]. This topic is presented in greater detail in Chapter 5.

DISCREPANT TRANSVAGINAL SONOGRAPHY AND BIOPSY RESULTS

We and others have observed several patients whose endometrial biopsies were negative, even though a definite sonographic abnormality was present[19]. Typically, this is the result of insufficient sampling, not a false-positive sonogram. The polyp is usually clearly apparent on transvaginal sonography and resampling, perhaps under transabdominal or transrectal guidance, may be used to definitely sample the abnormal area (Figure 3)[20].

TRANSVAGINAL COLOR DOPPLER SONOGRAPHY FINDINGS

Several studies have suggested that endometrial carcinoma is associated with increased vascularity within the endometrium, as well as a decreased impedance in the radial and uterine arteries. Focal areas of increased blood flow in a postmenopausal woman should be considered suspicious. Calculation of the impedance value in the blood vessels in the endometrium does not seem to differentiate benign from malignant entities, however[21].

SUMMARY

This chapter describes and illustrates the sonographic findings in endometrial cancer. Improved delineation of early cancer may be possible with the additional use of color Doppler sonography.

References

1. Osmers, R., Völksen, M. and Schauer, A. (1990). Vaginosonography for early detection of endometrial carcinoma? *Lancet,* **335**, 1569–71
2. Goldstein, S. R., Nachtigall, M., Snyder, J. R. *et al.* (1990). Endometrial assessment by vaginal ultrasonography before endometrial sampling in patients with postmenopausal bleeding. *Am. J. Obstet. Gynecol.,* **163**, 119
3. Schulman, H., Conway, C., Zalud, I., Farmakides, G., Haley, J. and Cassata, M. (1994). Prevalence in a volunteer population of pelvic cancer detected with transvaginal ultrasound and color flow Doppler. *Ultrasound Obstet. Gynecol.,* **4**, 414–20
4. Kurjak, A., Shalom, H. and Kupesic, S. (1994). Attempt to screen asymptomatic women for ovarian and endometrial cancer with transvaginal color and pulsed Doppler sonography. *J. Ultrasound Med.,* **13**(4), 295–7
5. Bourne, T. H. (1995). Evaluating the endometrium of postmenopausal women with transvaginal ultrasonography. *Ultrasound Obstet. Gynecol.,* **6**, 75–80

6. Holbert, T. R. (1994). Screening transvaginal ultrasonography of postmenopausal women in a private office setting. *Am. J. Obstet. Gynecol.,* **170,** 1699–704

7. Castelo-Branco, C., Puerto, B., Durán, M., Gratacós, E., Torné, A., Fortuny, A. and Vanrell, J. A. (1994). Transvaginal sonography of the endometrium in postmenopausal women: monitoring the effect of hormone replacement therapy. *Maturitas,* **19,** 59–65

8. Lin, M. C., Gosink, B. B., Wolfe, S. I. *et al.* (1991). Endometrial thickness after menopause: effect of hormone replacement. *Radiology,* **180,** 427–32

9. Levine, D., Goslick, B. and Johnson, L. (1995). Change in endometrial thickness in postmenopausal women undergoing hormone replacement therapy. *Radiology,* **197,** 603–8

10. Granberg, S., Wikland, M., Karlsson, B., Norström, A. and Friberg, L. G. (1991). Endometrial thickness as measured by endovaginal ultrasonography for identifying endometrial abnormality. *Am. J. Obstet. Gynecol.,* **164,** 47–52

11. Reinhold, C., Atri, M., Mehio, A., Zakarian, R., Aldis, A. E. and Bret, P. M. (1995). Diffuse uterine adenomyosis: morphologic criteria and diagnostic accuracy of endovaginal sonography. Radiology, **197,** 609–14

12. Cagnazzo, G., D'Addario, V., Martinelli, G. and Lastilla, G. (1992). Depth of myometrial invasion in endometrial cancer: preoperative assessment by transvaginal ultrasonography and magnetic resonance imaging. *Ultrasound Obstet. Gynecol.,* **2,** 40–3

13. Fedele, L., Bianchi, S., Dorta, M., Brioschi, D., Zanotti, F. and Vercellini, P. (1991). Transvaginal ultrasonography versus hysteroscopy in the diagnosis of uterine submucous myomas. *Obstet. Gynecol.,* **77,** 745–8

14. Huang, R-T., Chou, C-Y., Chang, C-H., Yu, C-H., Huang, S-C. and Yao, B-L. (1995). Differentiation between adenomyoma and leiomyoma with transvaginal ultrasonography. *Ultrasound Obstet. Gynecol.,* **5,** 47–50

15. Hirai, M., Shibata, K., Sagai, H., Sekiya, S. and Goldberg, B. B. (1995). Transvaginal pulsed and color Doppler sonography for the evaluation of adenomyosis. *J. Ultrasound Med.,* **14,** 529–32

16. Uzan, S., Perrot, N. and Uzan, M. (1993). Tamoxifen: vaginosonography and color Doppler assessment of the uterus. *Ultrasound Obstet. Gynecol.,* **3,** 305–6

17. Van Leeuwen, F. E., Benraadt, J., Coebergh, J. W. W., Kiemeney, L. A. L. M., Gimbrére, C. H. F., Otter, R., Schouten, L. J., Damhuis, R. A. M., Bontenbal, M., Diepenhorst, F. W., van den Belt-Dusebout, A. W. and van Tinteren, H. (1994). Risk of endometrial cancer after tamoxifen treatment of breast cancer. *Lancet,* **343,** 448–52

18. Dallenbach-Hellweg, G. and Hahn, U. (1995). Mucinous and clear cell adenocarcinomas of the endometrium in patients receiving antiestrogens (Tamoxifen) and gestagens. *Int. J. Gynecol. Pathol.,* **14,** 7–15

19. Dubinsky, T. J., Parvey, H. R., Gormaz, G., Curtis, M. and Maklad, N. (1995). Transvaginal hysterosonography: comparison with biopsy in the evaluation of postmenopausal bleeding. *J. Ultrasound Med.,* **14,** 887–93

20. Shipley, III C. F., Simmons, C. L. and Nelson, G. H. (1994). Comparison of transvaginal sonography with endometrial biopsy in asymptomatic postmenopausal women. *J. Ultrasound Med.,* **13,** 99–104

21. Sheth, S., Hamper, U. M., McCollum, M. E., Caskey, C. I., Rosenshein, N. B. and Kurman, R. J. (1995). Endometrial blood flow analysis in postmenopausal women: can it help differentiate benign from malignant causes of endometrial thickening? *Radiology,* **195,** 661–5

Transvaginal sonography of endometrium in fertility disorders

8

S. Kupesic and A. Kurjak

INTRODUCTION

The uterine cavity must provide an environment for successful sperm migration from the cervix to the Fallopian tube. The normality of the mucosal lining, glandular secretion and vascularity are necessary to support implantation and placentation. Uterine anomalies, polyps, myomata, neoplasia, infections and intrauterine scar tissue can lead to poor reproductive performance. Attempts have been made to correlate the sonographic parameters (such as thickness and reflectivity) and endometrial receptivity. This chapter emphasizes the role of transvaginal sonography and color Doppler imaging in evaluation of the endometrial function and detection of the endometrial abnormalities.

CONGENITAL ANOMALIES

A diagnosis of anatomic disorders is made in 38–55% of patients with recurrent pregnancy loss[1,2].

Sonographic identification of duplication anomalies of the uterus (such as septate uterus, bicornuate uterus, or uterus didelphyis) has the highest sensitivity and specificity during the secretory phase of the menstrual cycle. However, the accuracy of ultrasound for diagnosing the uterine anomalies depends on the severity of the anomaly[3]. During the secretory phase, the endometrium is most prominent: a separated echogenic line representing endometrium surrounded by hypoechoic myometrium and contour abnormality are easily identified (Figure 1). Conversely, a careful search with the transvaginal transducer may demonstrate a single uterine horn and atypical endometrial echo in a patient with uterus unicollis[4]. Large quantities of intra-cavitary fluid should raise the suspicion of an underlying obstruction in a case of imperforate hymen or vaginal atresia.

The use of continuous sonographic visualization for the assessment of the endometrial cavity during and after the instillation of the contrast fluid is called sonohysterography[5]. Using this method, uterine septa are precisely visualized and the extent of the septum can be delineated. In the hysterosonographic study of Randolph and co-workers[6], the results agreed with those of hysteroscopic examination in 53 out of 54 patients, yielding a sensitivity of 98% and specificity of 100%.

ENDOMETRIAL POLYP

Endometrial polyp is the anatomical defect that is implicated in the etiology of a recurrent pregnancy loss and infertility. Polyps appear as diffuse or focal thickening of the endometrium. Using sonohysterography, an intracavitary polyp is seen surrounded by anechoic fluid, with the point of the attachment[5]. If the examination is performed in the follicular phase, use of the distending medium is not necessary to detect abnormal endometrial thickening. However, during the periovulatory and secretory phase, polyps are better visualized when outlined by fluid.

By using transvaginal color and pulsed Doppler, we can study minor arteries supplying the growth of the endometrial polyp (Figures 2 and 3). For more information about color Doppler evaluation of the endometrial blood flow in this benign condition, see Chapter 9.

SUBMUCOUS FIBROIDS

The diagnosis of a submucous leiomyoma is based on distortion of the uterine contour, uterine enlargement and textural changes. Since leiomyomas have a varying amount of smooth muscle and connective tissue, these benign tumors also have a variety of sonographic features[6]. Sonographic texture ranges from hypoechoic to echogenic, depending on the amount of smooth muscle and connective tissue. Central ischemia, which is a consequence of tumor enlargement and inadequate blood supply, is usually followed by various stages of

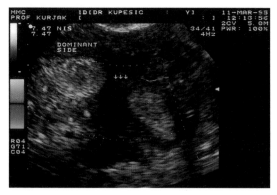

Figure 1 A transvaginal scan demonstrates duplication anomaly of the uterus. Note two separate endometria during the secretory phase of the menstrual cycle. Spiral arteries (left) are easily detected by color Doppler

degeneration. The most common cause of calcification within the uterus is calcific degeneration within a fibroid. Other types of degeneration include cystic, myxomatous and hyaline degeneration. Sometimes, because of the variety of appearances, submucous leiomyomas may be mistaken for endometrial polyps, endometrial carcinoma, blood, or mucus. Fedele and co-workers[7] evaluated the accuracy of transvaginal sonography in detection of small submucous myomas in patients who underwent both transvaginal ultrasound examination and hysteroscopy before hysterectomy. The sensitivity and specificity of transvaginal sonography were similar to those of hysteroscopy in that study.

In patients with submucous fibroids, the uterine environment is not conducive to nidation of a fertilized ovum and blood supply might be inadequate[8]. Deligdish and Loewenthal[9] performed a histological study of the endometrium at four sites in uteri containing submucous myomas. They found atrophy of the endometrial glands and stroma in the endometrium overlying or opposite the leiomyoma, while, at the border of the leiomyoma, hyperplastic glands were detected. This finding is secondary to increased vascularity and increased estrogen concentrations. Farrer-Brown and colleagues[10] were able to obtain vascular obstruction and venous dilatation within the overlying endometrium. Therefore, submucous leiomyoma may reduce

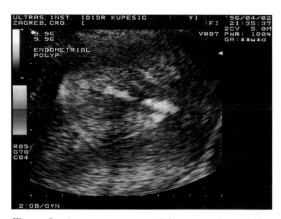

Figure 2 A transverse scan of the uterus in an infertile patient with irregular menstrual bleeding. Note the area of increased endometrial thickening representing a polyp. Regularly separated vessels are visualized by color Doppler

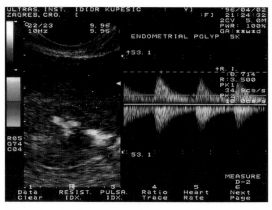

Figure 3 In the same patient as in Figure 2, color and pulsed Doppler indicate a benign uterine mass represented by the high resistance index (RI = 0.71)

blood flow, cause the progressive congestion and reduce the delivery of the hormones necessary for normal endometrial development. These changes can result in atrophy of the endometrium and inadequate placentation. Furthermore, submucous leiomyomas may interfere with expansion of the fetus or limit the compliance of the uterus[11].

Leiomyoma grows centripetally as proliferations of smooth muscle cells and fibrous connective tissue, creating a pseudocapsule of compressed muscle fibers. Therefore, color Doppler demonstrates most of the myometrial blood vessels at its periphery (Figures 4 and 5). The pre-

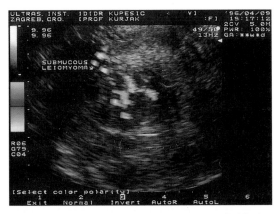

Figure 4 Submucous leiomyoma surrounded by hyperechoic endometrium. Color Doppler imaging demonstrates an increased vascularity at the base of the leiomyoma pedicle

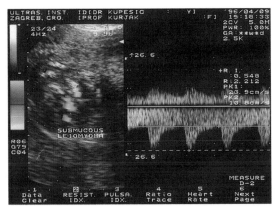

Figure 5 In the same patient as in Figure 4, color signals explored by pulsed Doppler waveform analysis (right) show moderate to high-resistance blood flow (RI = 0.55). The benign nature of the tumor was confirmed by histopathology

sence of blood vessels in the central portion of the leiomyomas is usually correlated with necrotic, degenerative and inflammatory changes. These vessels display lower resistance indices (RI) values than peripherally located vessels, and sometimes can be misinterpreted for malignant neovascular pulsed Doppler signal[12]. Vascular impedance to blood flow in myometrium supplying vessels depends not only on size but location within the uterus. A significant difference was shown in blood flow characteristics for leiomyoma-supplying vessels between entirely subserosal versus intramural and submucous leiomyomas. Lower impedance values for subserosal leiomyomas can be explained by the fact that these leiomyomas are supplied with blood vessels through a very small contact area. These blood vessels are surrounded with loose connective tissue and therefore dilated with very low vascular impedance to blood flow. In contrast, submucous leiomyomas and those located within the myometrium are supplied by blood vessels with higher vascular impedance. High basal tonus of myometrial tissue surrounding intramural or submucous leiomyomas could cause a difference in hemodynamic parameters.

Kurjak and colleagues[12] performed transvaginal color flow evaluation in 101 patients with palpable uterine fibroids and 60 healthy volunteers. The mean RI from the periphery of

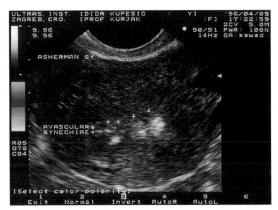

Figure 6 Transvaginal scan of a patient with intrauterine synechiae. Endometrial irregularities and avascular hyperechoic bridges are easily obtained

leiomyoma covered the value of 0.54. Mean pulsatility index (PI) value was 0.89. The pathohistological finding was benign uterine tumor in all the cases, even when RI was very low. Lowered RI were present in cases with necrosis and secondary degenerative and inflammatory changes within the fibroid. Increased blood flow velocity and decreased RI (mean RI = 0.74) in both uterine arteries occurred in patients with uterine fibroids.

ENDOMETRITIS

Chronic endometritis is characterized with increased echogenicity, thickness and vascularity of the endometrium[8]. The most common cause of chronic endometrial infection is *Mycobacterium tuberculosis*. During the activation of infection, pregnancy often terminates ectopically or as an abortion. Transvaginal sonographic findings may include calcified pelvic lymph nodes or smaller irregular calcifications in the adnexa, and deformity of the endometrial cavity suggestive of adhesions in the absence of a history of prior curettage or abortion. In the acute stage of the endometritis, low- to moderate-impedance blood flow signals are easily obtained on the periphery of the endometrium. On the contrary, blood flow is usually absent in cases with irreversible tissue damage. Transvaginal sonography allows elucidation of the abnormal endometrial morphology, after which appropriate cultures should be taken and broadspectrum antibiotic therapy administered. In order to prevent the development of intrauterine adhesions (especially after dilatation and curettage (D & C)), administration of conjugated estrogen for 1–2 months is recommended. This therapy allows regeneration of the healthy endometrium, which is paralleled by a sharp increase in end-diastolic velocities of the spiral arteries at the time of color flow and pulsed Doppler analysis.

ASHERMAN'S SYNDROME

In 1948, Asherman described eight cases of intrauterine stenosis[13]. Destruction of the endometrium may result in scarring and the development of bands of scar tissue, or synechiae, within the uterine cavity. This destruction may occur as a result of a vigorous curettage of the uterus following an abortion or, more often, after a curettage of an advanced pregnancy. Tuberculosis may also cause uterine synechiae, but only in rare cases. This may result in formation of adhesive bands of different size with a subsequent partial or total obliteration of the endometrial cavity. Menstrual pattern is characterized by amenorrhea or hypomenorrhea.

Patients with endometrial adhesion, such as Asherman's syndrome, may have a distorted endometrial pattern with areas where no endometrium can be imaged mixed with areas that appear normal[14]. Adhesions are observed as endometrial irregularities or hyperechoic bridges within the endometrial cavity (Figure 6).

Schlaff and Hurst[15] analyzed seven amenorrheic patients with severe Asherman's syndrome. Transvaginal sonography demonstrated a well-developed endometrial stripe in three of seven women, while three others had virtually no endometrium seen. All the patients with well-developed endometrium were found to have adhesions excluding the lower uterine segment and had resumption of normal menses and normalization of the cavity after hysteroscopy. The women with minimal endometrium had no cavity identified and derived no benefit from surgery. The conclusion of that study was that endometrial pattern on transvaginal sonography is highly predictive of both surgical and clinical outcome in patients with severe Asherman's syndrome characterized by complete obstruction of the cavity at hysterosalpingogram.

Intrauterine synechiae do not present increased vascularity on color Doppler examination. They are better visualized during menstruation when intracavitary fluid outlines them or following hysterosonography.

ENDOMETRIAL FACTORS IN INFERTILITY

Ultrasonographic examination is a non-invasive procedure and has the advantage that serial observation of the endometrial texture and thickness may be easily analyzed.

Endometrium which is the target organ for circulating estradiol and progesterone displays textural variations during the menstrual cycle. In the postmenstrual period, endometrium is visualized as a thin echogenic interface. In the proliferative phase, it becomes isoechoic in comparison with the myometrium. As ovulation approaches, the endometrium becomes more echogenic secondary to the development of secretions within the endometrial glands[3]. A hypoechoic halo probably arises from the inner layer of the myometrium, while a hypoechoic area within the endometrium results from edema of the compacta. During the secretory phase, a progressive increase of acoustic enhancement is observed as a result of progesterone action. This change of the endometrial pattern is due to the progressive increase of the mucous secretions and coiling phenomena of the endometrial glands. These events take place from the endometrial base towards the surface.

However, data on the use of sonography to interpret endometrial function are conflicting. Gonen and Casper[16] described three different types of the endometrial texture on the day of oocyte retrieval in an *in vitro* fertilization program. They found that triple-line endometrium was more likely to be associated with successful implantation than two other types (homogeneously hyperechoic or intermediate isoechogenic pattern). Furthermore, the endometrial thickness was greater in patients who become pregnant (8.7 ± 0.4 mm) than in the group who did not (7.5 ± 0.2 mm). Some publications[17–19] suggested that, in cases in which endometrial thickness was less than 6 mm, embryo implantation appeared drastically reduced. In contrast, when it exceeded 9 or 10 mm, optimal implantation rates were obtained. Smith and colleagues[20] felt that both endometrial thickness and pattern were important. Other investigators[21–23] have also analyzed the relationship between the endometrial thickness, texture and outcome and found statistically significant correlation.

Kepic and co-workers[24] determined that endometrial thickness and pattern, follicle size and estradiol levels correlated to both the likelihood of pregnancy and subsequent outcome.

Contrary to these data, studies of Fleischer and colleagues[25,26] found no correlation between endometrial thickness and embryo implantation.

Such conflicting results can be explained by the variability of the endometrial appearance according to the timing of the ultrasound scan (day of the human chorionic gonadotropin (hCG) administration, day of the oocyte pick-up or day of the embryo transfer). It seems that the most promising data were obtained when the study was performed on the day of hCG administration, since the progesterone production does not interfere with endometrial characteristics at this period of the menstrual cycle. Li and colleagues[27] examined the prevalence of abnormal endometrial development during the luteal phase of infertile ($n = 142$) and fertile ($n = 68$) populations. The authors have used histological dating by traditional criteria. The prevalence of a retarded endometrium was significantly higher in the infertile than in the control group (14% versus 4.4%).

The authors subdivided the infertile patients into four subgroups (according to the cause of infertility). Patients suffering from endometriosis had a significantly higher prevalence (29%) of abnormal endometrial development, while no difference occurred in patients with tubal or male infertility. Furthermore, 21% of patients with unexplained infertility had out-of-phase endometrium. Summarized results are presented in Table 1.

Further technological development resulted in a combination of transvaginal color and pulsed Doppler with real-time sonography. This method proposed to obtain a valuable information concerning the uterine receptivity by studying the uterine artery perfusion. Furthermore, the impedance indices of the uterine artery were found to be predictive of a pregnancy outcome[28–30].

The blood supply to the endometrium is derived from the branches of the uterine arteries. Radial arteries extend through the myometrium and form two types of terminal branches: straight and coiled (Figure 7).

The straight branches, called basal arteries, supply the basalis layer of the endometrium. The coiled branches, called spiral arteries, traverse the endometrium and supply the functionalis layer[31].

The spiral arteries, like the endometrium and unlike the basal arteries, are remarkably responsive to the hormonal changes during the menstrual cycle (Figure 8).

Kupesic and Kurjak[32] were first to report spiral artery perfusion during the periovulatory period in spontaneous and induced ovarian cycles with both sonographically and hormonally confirmed ovulation. Increased blood flow velocity and decreased spiral artery impedance occurred the day before ovulation in the group with spontaneous cycles (PI = 1.13) compared with the hormonally stimulated group (PI = 2.32). Endometrial thickness was significantly decreased in patients in whom

Table 1 A comparison of the age, duration of infertility, follicular phase length, luteal phase length, and the prevalence of retarded endometrial development among four groups of infertile subjects and a group of normal fertile subjects

	Group I (tubal) (n = 34)	Group II (male) (n = 21)	Group III (endometriosis) (n = 48)	Group IV (unexplained) (n = 48)	Group V (normal) (n = 68)
Age (years)	32.5 ± 4.0 (NS)	30.8 ± 4.0 (NS)	34.0 ± 2.9 (NS)	32.7 ± 4.4 (NS)	33.4 ± 4.0
Duration of infertility (years)	6.1 ± 3.3 (NS)	6.8 ± 2.7 (NS)	6.9 ± 2.9 (NS)	6.0 ± 3.3 (NS)	—
Follicular phase length (days)	14.3 ± 3.2 (NS)	13.7 ± 2.1 (NS)	13.9 ± 2.1 (NS)	14.5 ± 2.4 (NS)	13.6 ± 1.8
Luteal phase length (days)	13.2 ± 1.0 (NS)	13.1 ± 1.6 (NS)	11.9 ± 1.5 (NS)	12.7 ± 1.8 (NS)	12.9 ± 1.5
Prevalence of retarded endometrium (histologic dating by traditional criteria), $n/n(\%)$	1/34(2.9) (NS)	3/39(7.7) (NS)	6/21(29) ($p < 0.01$)	10/48(21) ($p < 0.01$)	3/68(4.4)

From Li and co-workers[27], with permission; the results (with the exception of the prevalence of retarded endometrium) shown are mean ± SD. The results in the four groups of infertile subjects are compared individually to the normal fertile subjects by two-sample t-tests or 2×2 contingency table analysis. NS, not significant

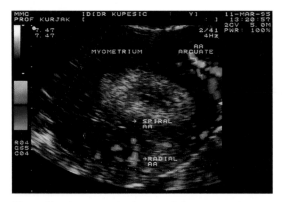

Figure 7 A transvaginal scan of the uterus demonstrating arcuate artery network, radial arteries extending through the myometrium and spiral arteries at the periphery of the endometrium

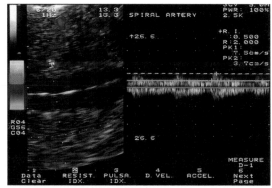

Figure 8 Color signals obtained from the spiral arteries on the periphery of the multi-layered endometrium. Blood flow velocity waveforms obtained during the periovulatory period demonstrate decreased resistance index (RI = 0.50)

Table 2 Endometrial thickness (in mm) during 27 spontaneous and 51 induced cycles. Values are means ± SD

		Days before and after ovulation				
	n	−3	−2	−1	0	+1
Spontaneous cycles	27	8 ± 1.1	10 ± 1.2	12 ± 1.4	12 ± 1.5	13 ± 1.2
Induced cycles						
CC (first cycle)	15	7 ± 1.5	9 ± 1.4	11 ± 1.4	12 ± 1.2	13 ± 1.6
CC[†] (subsequent cycles)	12	4 ± 1.5	6 ± 2.0	7 ± 2.0	7 ± 1.8	7 ± 2.0
CC/hMG	16	5 ± 1.5	6 ± 2.0	8 ± 2.0	9 ± 2.5	9 ± 2.0
HMG	8	6 ± 1.8	8 ± 2.0	11 ± 1.8	12 ± 2.0	12 ± 1.8

From Kupesic and Kurjak[32] with permission; [†]Ovulation; CC, clomiphene citrate; hMG, human menopausal gonadotropin

clomiphene citrate (CC) was used for follicular stimulation for three or more times compared with spontaneous and first CC-stimulated cycles (Table 2). Significantly thicker endometrium was observed in human menopausal gonadotropin (hMG)-stimulated patients compared with the CC/hMG group throughout the follicular phase of the cycle. Clear flow velocity waveforms were obtained from 80% of the endometria of the patients stimulated for the first time with CC. On the contrary, spiral artery perfusion was detected and evaluated on a daily basis only in 16.7% of patients with CC stimulation or three or more cycles. Analyzing the spiral artery blood flow regarding to the type of stimulation, significant difference ($p < 0.001$) occurred in the CC/hMG-stimulated group compared with others (Figure 9).

Clomiphene citrate is shown to deplete estrogen (E) receptors in E-sensitive tissue influencing both endometrial growth and pattern[33–36].

Kupesic and Kurjak[32] found a strong correlation between endometrial thickness and flow velocities. However, this does not apply to the group of patients stimulated with CC/hMG and normal endometrial growth where absence of diastolic flow was detected in 55.6% of patients.

Zaidi and colleagues[37] analyzed endometrial thickness, endometrial morphology and presence or absence of subendometrial or intra-endometrial color flow in 96 infertile patients undergoing *in vitro* fertilization treatment. The results of the study obtained on the day of hCG administration were related to the pregnancy rates. The overall pregnancy rate was 32.3% and

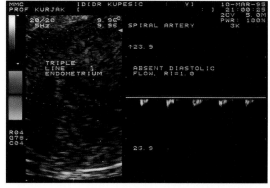

Figure 9 Blood flow velocity waveforms of the spiral arteries obtained from the triple-line endometrium (left). The absence of the diastolic flow is a sign of poor endometrial perfusion (right) and correlates with poor endometrial receptivity

there was no significant difference between pregnant and non-pregnant groups with regard to endometrial thickness. The pregnancy rates were not significantly different for different endometrial morphological patterns ($p > 0.05$). The absence of endometrial blood flow was associated with the failure of implantation ($p < 0.05$). However, no difference in pregnancy rates was found related to the zones of vascular penetration (subendometrial, outer hyperechogenic zone, or inner hypoechogenic zone).

Both studies analyzing endometrial blood flow reported that color and pulsed Doppler can be used to monitor the uterine receptivity and to reveal unexplained infertility problems.

Another problem of clinical importance is luteal phase defect. This is defined as a lack of more than 2 days in a histological development of the endometrium compared to the day of the cycle[38,39]. Several methods have been developed to evaluate endometrial function, such as quantitative histology, electron microscopy, histochemistry and immunohistochemistry, hysteroscopy and measurement of endometrial protein levels in plasma or endometrial washing. All the methods mentioned are invasive and cause some discomfort to the patient and could potentially interrupt implantation in a conception cycle. Therefore, Doherty and co-workers used transvaginal sonography for the assessment of luteal phase endometrium and non-invasive identification of patients with luteal phase defect[40].

A recent Doppler study was undertaken in an attempt to establish a relationship between the color Doppler analysis of the segmental uterine and ovarian circulation and histological dating on the endometrial biopsy[41]. Spiral arteries in the control group demonstrated RI of 0.53 ± 0.04 during the periovulatory phase, while RI of 0.50 ± 0.02 and 0.51 ± 0.04 were obtained during the midluteal and late luteal phases, respectively. Higher impedance values during the periovulatory (RI = 0.70 ± 0.06, $p < 0.001$), mid-luteal phase (RI = 0.72 ± 0.06, $p < 0.001$) and late luteal phase (RI = 0.72 ± 0.04, $p < 0.001$) were obtained from the spiral arteries in the luteal phase defect group. Data on ovarian and intraovarian vascular impedance demonstrated significant differences between the normal and the luteal phase defect group.

Therefore, color and pulsed Doppler analysis of the corpus luteum and minor endometrial vessels may aid in assessing the luteal phase adequacy.

AGE AND ENDOMETRIAL FACTOR

The groups of Navot[42] and Edwards[43] addressed the relationship of increasing maternal age and decline in fertility. Both studies found that amenorrheic women or patients over the age of 40 who received donor oocytes had better implantation and pregnancy rates than those who were cycling but received their own oocytes.

Therefore, the main determinant of reproductive outcome in this age group is oocyte quality rather than endometrial receptivity. Decline in fertility potential may be readily restored by oocyte donation in an artificially induced cycle. Recent studies by Batista and colleagues[44] proved normal luteal and endometrial secretory function and normal endometrial maturation in cycling women over 40 years. Their results clearly indicate that implantation failure due to a hostile endometrium does not play a significant role in the decline of fertility in this population.

Kurjak and Kupesic[45] performed serial measurements throughout the menstrual cycle in 120 normal cycling women with documented infertility, 85 postmenopausal patients and 45 postmenopausal patients receiving hormone replacement therapy. They found obvious changes in the flow velocity patterns of the ovarian, uterine, radial and spiral arteries with age. The fact that the uterine artery RI did not change significantly in the first postmenopausal years strongly supports the thesis that the aging process initially affects the uterus less than the ovary. Furthermore, the uterine environment could be easily manipulated during the menopausal years by proper hormonal stimulation.

ENDOMETRIAL PERISTALSIS

Birnholtz[46] was first to report endometrial movements as a reflection of the myometrial activity. These contractions are most common in the follicular phase and culminate around ovulation. At that time the contractions are towards the fundus and may help the sperm transport and maintenance of pregnancy. However, first observations have been done by transabdominal ultrasound and quantification of the movement was not attempted.

Oike and co-workers[47] used transvaginal sonography to obtain endometrial movements in the proliferative phase of the menstrual cycle, while they were not able to detect any contractility during the secretory phase of the menstrual cycle. In 1990 Abramowitz and Archer[48] and De Vries and colleagues[49] made a classification of the movements in terms of intensity and frequency using the transvaginal probe. The ideal method to observe this peristaltic motion is by recording the examination on the video tape and later playing back the tape at accelerated speed. De Vries and colleagues performed 46 examinations on 42 consecutive women. The authors stated that contractions were retrograde in all phases of the menstrual cycles except during the menstruation. The same statements have been proved by Lyons and co-workers in 1991[50].

Oike and colleagues[51] correlated endometrial activity with hormonal levels. They found that endometrial peristalsis had a strong correlation to estradiol levels. Rising progesterone levels seemed to reduce the frequency of endometrial/myometrial movements. Preliminary data of Abramowitz and Archer suggest that the disturbance of peristaltic contraction may play a role in some cases of unexplained infertility.

References

1. Kutteh, W. and Carr, B. (1993). Recurrent pregnancy loss. In *Textbook of Reproductive Medicine*, pp. 559–70. (Norwalk: Appleton and Lange)

2. Stray-Pedersen, B. and Stray-Pedersen, S. (1984). Etiological factors and subsequent reproductive performance in 195 couples with a prior history of habitual abortion. *Am. J. Obstet. Gynecol.*, **148**, 140–6

3. Fleischer, A. C. and Keppe, D. M. (1992). Benign conditions of the uterus, cervix and endometrium. In Nyberg, A., Hill, L. M., Bohm-Velez, M. and Mendelson, E. B. (eds.) *Transvaginal Ultrasound*, pp. 21–43. (St Louis: Mosby Year Book)

4. Funk, A. and Fendel, H. (1988). Sonography diagnosis of congenital uterine abnormalities. *Z. Geburtshilfe Perinatol.*, **192**, 77–88

5. Cullinan, J. A., Fleischer, A. C., Kepple, D. M. and Aenoco, A. L. (1995). Sonohysterography: a technique for endometrial evaluation. *Radiographics*, **15**, 501–14

6. Randolph, J. R., Ying, Y. K., Maier, D. B., Schmidt, C. L. and Riddick, D. H. (1986). Comparison of real-time ultrasonography, hysterosalpingography and laparotomy/hysteroscopy in the evaluation of the uterine abnormalities and tubal patency. *Fertil. Steril.*, **46**, 828–32

7. Fedele, L., Bianchi, S. and Dorta, M. (1991). Transvaginal ultrasonography versus hysteroscopy in the diagnosis of uterine submocous myomas. *Obstet. Gynecol.*, **77**, 745–8

8. Kurjak, A. and Kupesic, S. (1994). Benign uterine conditions. In Kurjak, A. (ed.) *An Atlas of Transvaginal Color Doppler*, pp. 247–317. (Carnforth, UK: Parthenon Publishing)

9. Deligdish, L. and Loewenthal, M. (1970). Endometrial changes associated with myomata of the uterus. *J. Clin. Pathol.*, **23**, 676

10. Farrer-Brown, G., Beilby, J. O. and Tarbit, M. H. (1971). Venous changes in the endometrium of myomatous uteri. *Obstet. Gynecol.*, **38**, 743

11. Winkel, A. C. (1993). Diagnosis and treatment of uterine pathology. In Carr, B. R. and Blackwell, R. E. (eds.) *Textbook of Reproductive Medicine*, pp. 481–505. (Norwalk: Appleton and Lange)

12. Kurjak, A., Kupesic, S. and Miric, D. (1992). The assessment of benign uterine tumor vascularization by transvaginal color Doppler. *Ultrasound Med. Biol.*, **18**, 645–9

13. Asherman, J. G. (1948). Amenorrhea traumatica (atretica). *J. Obstet. Gynaecol. Br. Emp.*, **55**, 23

14. Dodson, M. (1995). The endometrium. In Dodson, M. (ed.) *Transvaginal Ultrasound*, pp. 73–103. (New York: Churchill Livingstone)

15. Schlaff, W. D. and Hurst, B. S. (1995). Preoperative sonographic measurement of endometrial pattern predicts outcome of surgical repair in patients with severe Asherman's syndrome. *Fertil. Steril.*, **63**, 410–3

16. Gonen, Y. and Casper, R. F. (1990). Prediction of implantation by the sonographic appearance of the endometrium during controlled ovarian stimulation for *in vitro* fertilization. *J. In Vitro Fertil. Embryo Transfer*, **7**, 146–52

17. Dickey, R. P., Olar, T. T., Curole, D. N., Taylor, S. N. and Rye, P. H. (1992). Endometrial pattern and thickness associated with pregnancy outcome after assisted reproduction technologies. *Hum. Reprod.*, **7**, 418–21

18. Sher, G., Herbert, C., Massarani, G. and Jacobs, M. H. (1991). Assessment of the undergoing IVF-ET. *Hum. Reprod.*, **6**, 232–7

19. Glissant, A., de Mouzon, J. and Frydman, R. (1985). Ultrasound study of the endometrium during IVF cycles. *Fertil. Steril.*, **44**, 786–90

20. Smith, B., Porter, R., Ahuja, K. and Craft, I. (1984). Ultrasonic assessment of endometrial changes in stimulated cycles in an *in vitro* fertilization and embryo transfer program. *J. In Vitro Fertil. Embryo Transfer*, **1**, 233–8

21. Rabinowitz, R., Laufer, N., Lewin, A. *et al.* (1986). The value of ultrasonographic endometrial measurement in the prediction of pregnancy following *in vitro* fertilization. *Fertil. Steril.*, **45**, 824–8

22. Welker, B. G., Dembruch, U., Diedrich, K., Al-Hasani, S. and Krebs, D. (1989). TVS of the endometrium during oocyte pick-up in stimulated cycles for IVF. *J. Ultrasound Med.*, **1**, 233–8

23. Thickman, D., Arger, P., Turek, R., Biasco, L., Mintz, M. and Coleman, B. (1986). Sonographic assessment of the endometrium in patients undergoing *in vitro* fertilization. *J. Ultrasound Med.*, **5**, 197–210

24. Kepic, T., Applebaum, M. and Valle, J. (1992). Preovulatory follicular size, endometrial appearance, and estradiol levels in both conception and non-conception cycles: a retrospective study, 40th Annual Clinical Meeting of the American College of Obstetricians and Gynecologists, April: 20 (abstract)

25. Fleischer, A. C., Herbert, C. M., Sacks, G. A., Wentz, A. C., Entman, S. S. and James, A. E. Jr. (1986). Sonography of the endometrium during conception and non-conception cycles of *in vitro* fertilization and embryo transfer. *Fertil. Steril.*, **46**, 442–7

26. Fleischer, A. C., Pittaway, O., Beard, L., Thieme, G., Bundy, A., James, A. and Weritz, A. (1984). Sonographic depletion of endometrial changes occurring with ovulation induction. *J. Ultrasound Med.*, **3**, 341–2

27. Li, T. C., Dockery, P. and Cooke, I. D. (1991). Endometrial development in the luteal phase of women with various types of infertility: comparison with women of normal fertility. *Hum. Reprod.*, **6**, 325–30

28. Sterzik, K., Grab, D., Sasse, V., Hutter, W., Rosenbusch, B. and Terinde, R. (1989). Doppler sonographic findings and their correlation with implantation in an *in vitro* fertilization program. *Fertil. Steril.*, **52**, 825–8

29. Steer, C. V., Campbell, S., Tan, S. L., Crayford, T., Mills, C., Mason, B. A. and Collins, W. P. (1992). The use of transvaginal color flow imaging after *in vitro* fertilization to identify optimum uterine conditions before embryo transfer. *Fertil. Steril.*, **57**, 372–6

30. Bassil, S., Magritte, J. P., Roth, J., Nisolle, M., Donnez, J. and Gordts, S. (1995). Uterine vascularity during stimulation and its correlation with implantation in *in-vitro* fertilization. *Hum. Reprod.*, **6**, 1497–501

31. Applebaum, M. (1995). The menstrual cycle, menopause, ovulation induction, and *in vitro* fertilization. In Copel, J. A. and Reed, K. L. (eds.) *Doppler Ultrasound in Obstetrics and Gynecology*, pp. 71–86. (New York: Raven Press Ltd)

32. Kupesic, S. and Kurjak, A. (1993). Uterine and ovarian perfusion during the periovulatory period assessed by transvaginal color Doppler. *Fertil. Steril.*, **60**, 439–43

33. Aksel, S., Saracoglu, O. F., Yeoman, R. R. and Wiebe, R. H. (1986). Effects of the clomiphene citrate on cytosolic estradiol and progesterone receptor concentrations in secretory endometrium. *Am. J. Obstet. Gynecol.*, **155**, 1219–23

34. Wolman, I., Sagi, J., Pauzner, D., Yove, I., Seidman, D. S. and David, M. P. (1994). Transabdominal ultrasonographic evaluation of endometrial thickness in clomiphene citrate-stimulated cycles in relation to conception. *J. Clin. Ultrasound*, **22**, 109–12

35. Check, J. H., Dieterich, C. and Lurie, D. (1995). The effect of consecutive cycles of clomiphene citrate therapy on endometrial thickness and echo pattern. *Obstet. Gynecol.*, **86**, 341–5

36. Yagel, S., Ben-Chetrit, A., Anteby, E., Zacut, D., Hochner-Celnikier, D. and Ron, M. (1992). The effect of ethynil estradiol on endometrial thickness and uterine volume during ovulation induction by clomiphene citrate. *Fertil. Steril.*, **57**, 33–6

37. Zaidi, J., Campbell, S., Pittrof, R. and Tan, S. L. (1995). Endometrial thickness, morphology, vascular penetration and velocimetry in predicting implantation in an *in vitro* fertilization program. *Ultrasound Obstet. Gynecol.*, **6**, 191–8

38. Noyes, R. W., Hertig, A. T. and Rock, J. (1950). Dating the endometrial biopsy. *Fertil. Steril.*, **1**, 3–25

39. Dawood, Y. M. (1994). Corpus luteum insufficiency. *Curr. Opin. Obstet. Gynecol.*, **6**, 121–7

40. Doherty, C. M., Silver, B., Binor, Z., Wood Molo, M. and Radwanska, E. (1993). Transvaginal ultrasonography and the assessment of luteal phase endometrium. *Am. J. Obstet. Gynecol.*, **168**, 1702–9

41. Kupesic, S., Kurjak, A., Vujisic, S. and Petrovic, Z. (1997). Luteal phase defect; comparison between Doppler velocimetry, histological and hormonal markers. *Ultrasound Obstet. Gynecol.*, **9**, 105–12

42. Navot, D., Bergh, P. A., Williams, M. A., Garrisi, G. J., Guzman, I., Sander, B. and Grunfeld, L. (1991). Poor oocyte quality rather than implantation failure as a cause of age-related decline in female fertility. *Lancet*, **337**, 1375–7

43. Edwards, R. G., Morcos, S., MacNamee, M., Balamaceda, J. P., Walters, D. E. and Asch, R. (1991). High fecundity of amenorrhoeic women

in embryo-transfer programmes. *Lancet*, **338**, 292–4

44. Batista, M., Cartledge, T. P., Zellmer, A. M., Merimo, M. J., Axiotis, C., Bremner, N. J. and Nieman, L. K. (1995). Effects of aging on menstrual cycle hormones and endometrial maturation. *Fertil. Steril.*, **64**, 492–9

45. Kurjak, A. and Kupesic, S. (1995). Ovarian senescence and its significance on uterine and ovarian perfusion. *Fertil. Steril.*, **64**, 532–7

46. Birnholtz, J. (1984). Ultrasonographic visualization of endometrial movements. *Fertil. Steril.*, **41**, 157–8

47. Oike, K., Obata, S., Tagaki, K., Matsuo, K., Ishihan, K. and Kikuchi, S. (1988). Observation of endometrial movements with transvaginal sonography. *J. Ultrasound Med.*, **7**, 899

48. Abramowitz, J. S. and Archer, D. F. (1990). Uterine endometrial peristalsis – a transvaginal ultrasound study. *Fertil. Steril.*, **54**, 4512–14

49. De Vries, K., Lyons, F. A., Ballard, G., Levi, C. S. and Lindsay, D. J. (1990). Contractions of the inner third of the myometrium. *Am. J. Obstet. Gynecol.*, **162**, 679–82

50. Lyons, E. A., Ballard, G., Taylor, P. H., Levi, C. S., Zhieng, X. H. and Kredentser, J. V. (1991). Characterization of subendometrial myometrial contractions throughout the menstrual cycle in normal fertile women. *Fertil. Steril.*, **55**, 771–4

51. Oike, K., Ishihara, K. and Kikuchi, S. (1990). A study of the endometrial movement and serum hormonal level in connection with uterine contraction. *Acta Obstet. Gynecol. Jpn.*, **42**, 86–92

Color Doppler assessment of endometrial blood flow

9

A. Kurjak, S. Kupesic and M. M. Babic

INTRODUCTION

Assessment of the female pelvis is greatly facilitated by color Doppler imaging that allows for simultaneous overlayed display of anatomic (gray-scale) and flow (color) information[1]. Transvaginal color Doppler affords detailed delineation of the uterus and its myometrium, endometrium and vessels[2].

The vascular supply to the uterus is provided by a complex network of arteries originating from the uterine artery. Its main branches extend inward for about a third of the endometrium, forming the arcuate wreath which encircles the uterus[3]. Smaller branches called radial arteries are directed towards the uterine lumen. When passing the inner third of the myometrium and myometrial–endometrial junction they become spiral arteries. Endometrium appears as an echogenic interface in the central part of the uterus and transvaginal sonography permits its detailed delineation[4]. Endometrial thickness and texture are highly dependent on the concentration of circulating estrogen and progesterone. By using transvaginal color Doppler, it becomes possible to study the alterations of endometrial perfusion under physiological and pathophysiological conditions.

ADENOMYOSIS

Adenomyosis of the uterus is a condition in which clusters of endometrial tissue occur deep within the myometrium. It may be localized immediately adjacent to the endometrium, or it may extend through the myometrium, and even penetrate the serosa.

Most patients with adenomyosis have either a normal-sized uterus or non-specific findings of uterine enlargement[5]. A diffusely enlarged uterus with a thickened, 'Swiss cheese' appearance of the myometrium due to areas of hemorrhage and clots within the muscle has been reported as an appearance suggestive of adenomyosis[6] (Figure 1). Disordered echogenicity of the middle layer of the myometrium is usually present in severe cases. Sometimes the uterus is generally hypoechoic, while the large cysts are rarely seen. The most common symptoms are dysmenorrhea and hypermenorrhea. Significant pain during menstruation is caused by bleeding of the endometrial tissue within the muscle of the uterus. If performed, hysterosalpingography may demonstrate contrast medium penetrating into the myometrium.

Using transvaginal color Doppler and spectral analysis, it becomes possible to study uterine vascularity in this benign condition and to compare it with perfusion in other benign lesions. The mean resistance index (RI) of the flow detected within the myometrium was 0.56, while the RI of the uterine arteries showed a decreased value, such as 0.75 when compared to healthy volunteers (RI = 0.87) (Figure 2). Some of the difference between myoma and adenomyoma may be explained by the fact that estrogen receptors are found in higher concentrations in myoma than in the surrounding myometrium and leiomyomas are responsive to the variations of the luteal hormone[7], while adenomyosis cases have been demonstrated to lack estrogen and progesterone receptors[8]. Therefore, variations of hormones may have little effect on adenomyosis.

Hirai and colleagues[9] examined 44 benign uterine masses and seven uterine malignancies. They used transvaginal color and pulsed Doppler imaging to determine whether this technique is useful to differentiate adenomyosis from uterine malignancies. The authors also made a scoring system for diagnosis of adenomyosis. Their scoring system consisted of myometrial thickness, myometrial texture, contour and color Doppler analysis. The RI tended to be lower for uterine malignancies (mean $RI = 0.40 \pm 0.07$) as opposed to adenomyosis (mean $RI = 0.57 \pm 0.08$). The RI for myoma was almost the same as that for adenomyosis (mean $RI = 0.57$). The maximal velocity (V_{max}) tended to be higher for uterine malignancies than for adenomyosis. The V_{max} for myoma was slightly higher than that for adenomyosis. The conclusion is that a statistically significant difference exists between adenomyosis and uterine malignancies in both RI and V_{max}. However, no significant differences were noted between adenomyosis and myoma in RI and only slight differences were seen in V_{max}.

ENDOMETRITIS

Endometritis may produce increased thickness, echogenicity and vascularity of the endometrium and inner third of the myometrium. The waveforms detected from such color-coded areas show a moderately high resistance index (RI > 0.50) (Figure 3).

DECIDUA

When the uterine cavity is empty, showing a decidual reaction, or only a weak central fluid ring, a suspicion of ectopic pregnancy must be aroused if the pregnancy test is positive. The specific ultrasonic demonstration of ectopic

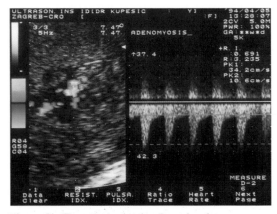

Figure 1 Color flow indicating a diffuse uterine blood flow and 'Swiss cheese' appearance of the myometrium in a patient suffering from adenomyosis

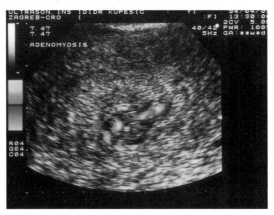

Figure 2 Transvaginal color Doppler demonstrates disordered echogenicity of the proximal layer of the myometrium in a patient with adenomyosis (left). Waveform analysis (right) shows moderate velocity and high-resistance blood flow (RI = 0.69)

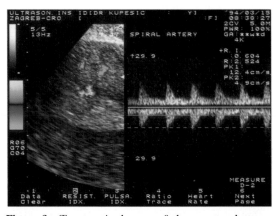

Figure 3 Transvaginal scan of the uterus demonstrating increased thickness, echogenicity and vascularity of the endometrium and inner third of the myometrium in a patient suffering from endometritis (left). Moderate-to-high impedance to blood flow (RI = 0.60) was isolated from the interrogated vessels

pregnancy is limited to cases with clear visualization of a living embryo or gestational ring outside the uterus[1]. When a non-specific complex adnexal mass is present, transvaginal color Doppler seems to be helpful in demonstrating low-impedance flow on the side of an ectopic pregnancy. In contrast to two concentric rings of decidua identified in early intrauterine pregnancy, the decidual ring associated with ectopic pregnancy has only one layer of decidua. Jurkovic and colleagues[10] compared the vascular signature in these two conditions. They

found that blood flow impedances in uterine and spiral arteries (Figure 4), and in corpus luteum blood vessels show no significant difference between intrauterine and ectopic pregnancies. The peak systolic velocity in the uterine arteries was the parameter which precisely reflected a decreased blood supply to the ectopic pregnancy. Transvaginal color Doppler is essential for analysis of the vascular supply to an ectopic pregnancy and selection of patients for conservative, non-interventional treatment.

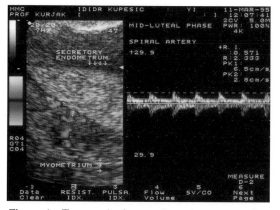

Figure 4 Transvaginal scan of an empty uterus in a case of suspected ectopic pregnancy and subnormal level of β-human chorionic gonadotropin. Moderate-impedance blood flow signals (RI = 0.57) are detected from the periphery of the thickened and homogeneously hyperechoic endometrium

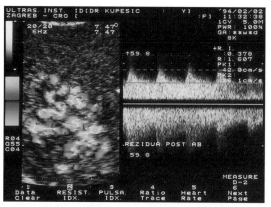

Figure 5 Transvaginal scan of the uterus containing retained products of conception. Color flow imaging accurately demonstrates low-impedance blood flow signals (RI = 0.38) typical of trophoblastic tissue

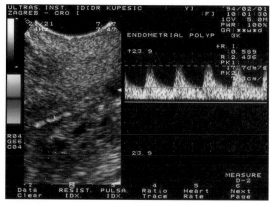

Figure 6 Transvaginal color Doppler demonstrating vascularized endometrial polyp (left). Pulsed Doppler waveform analysis (right) and RI of 0.59 indicate the benign nature of this endometrial structure

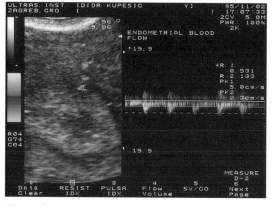

Figure 7 Doppler signals obtained from thick and hyperechoic endometrium in a perimenopausal patient demonstrating moderate impedance to blood flow (RI = 0.53). Endometrial hyperplasia was confirmed by histopathology

INCOMPLETE ABORTION

Transvaginal sonography has markedly reduced the uncertainties in diagnosis of early pregnancy failures. The diagnostic capacity of color Doppler ultrasound and its value as a predictor of pregnancy outcome are still unclear. No differences were observed in the blood flow velocity waveforms of uteroplacental vessels between uncomplicated early pregnancies and those which miscarried[11]. On the other hand, some studies mentioned a marked rate of decrease in RI in patients with spontaneous abortion and anembryonic pregnancy[11,12]. An abnormal flow pattern, such as continuous intervillous flow before 12 weeks of gestation in cases of missed abortion and blighted ovum, has to be studied in detail. The color Doppler is potentially valuable in the detection of abnormal hemochorial placentation and may greatly improve our understanding of early pregnancy failure. By this method, it becomes possible to detect changes in uterine perfusion in cases of incomplete abortion even without clear viability of the products of conception.

Incomplete abortions vary with the stage of embryological development at the time of the demise and the amount of gestational tissue passed. Variable amounts of disorganized echogenic debris, fluid, or both are often present in the endometrial cavity. Transvaginal color Doppler demonstrates rich perfusion of the unexpelled gestational tissue (Figure 5). Abundant color flow is caused by the dilated spiral arteries and venous system, probably in response to the active trophoblastic tissue.

ENDOMETRIAL POLYPS

Endometrial polyps develop as solitary or multiple soft, sessile and pedunculated tumors often composed of hyperplastic endometrium[1,2]. Approximately two-thirds contain no functional endometrium, and they often display a microscopic picture of cystic hyperplasia. The vascularization of endometrial polyps is supported by already existing vessels originating from terminal branches of the uterine arteries (Figure 6).

Sometimes polyps are necrotic and inflamed, and in these cases it is possible to identify flow in regularly separated vessels and analyze the velocity of blood flow through them[1]. The diastolic flow is always present, and the RI is usually higher than 0.45. A marked reduction in blood flow impedance noted on the periphery and/or within the endometrial polyps may lead an inexperienced ultrasonographer to false-positive diagnosis of endometrial malignancy.

ENDOMETRIAL HYPERPLASIA

Abnormal endometrial thickness may be present in some other benign uterine conditions such as endometrial hyperplasia. Endometrial thickness greater than 14 mm in premenopausal, and greater than 8 mm in postmenopausal women should be an indicator for further investigation[1]. The peak incidence of adenomatous hyperplasia is between 40 and 50 years of age. The sonographic findings have to be interpreted in light of the patient's clinical presentation and laboratory findings. Morphology itself cannot be used to discriminate benign from malignant conditions. Color and pulsed Doppler features serve as additional discriminative criteria for more accurate diagnosis of endometrial pathology[1,15]. The peripheral distribution of the regularly separated vessels is typical of endometrial hyperplasia (Figure 7). Color flow and pulsed Doppler signals are usually obtained from the border of the hyperplastic endometrium. A significant difference has been found in terms of the RI value between endometrial malignancy (mean RI = 0.42) and endometrial hyperplasia (mean RI = 0.50).

ENDOMETRIAL CARCINOMA

The problem of differentiating endometrial hyperplasia from carcinoma (both have a thick endometrium) is still unsolved by B-mode transvaginal sonography alone.

Angiogenesis is required for both tumor growth and progression, and is regarded as one of the most important events occurring in the neoplastic process. In a recent paper, Abulafia and co-workers[13] evaluated angiogenesis in endometrial hyperplasia and stage I endometrial carcinoma, as well as the relationship between angiogenesis and tumor grade and depth of invasion. Three groups of patients were analyzed: control patients who underwent hysterectomy for benign conditions ($n = 19$), patients with endometrial hyperplasia ($n = 24$), and patients with stage I endometrial carcinoma ($n = 34$). All hysterectomy specimens were stained immunohistochemically for factor VIII-related antigen as a sensitive and specific marker for vascular endothelium. Areas close to deepest myometrial invasion or those with the highest grade of endometrial hyperplasia and the highest angiogenic intensity were selected. Their study demonstrated increased angiogenicity of complex endometrial hyperplasia compared with controls or simple hyperplasia; similar angiogenic capability of complex hyperplasia compared with stage IA endometrial carcinoma; increased angiogenesis in invasive (stages IB and IC) endometrial carcinoma compared with complex hyperplasia or stage IA endometrial carcinoma; and increasing angiogenesis with higher tumor grade. Because of the limited number of patients within each subgroup of stage IB and IC endometrial carcinoma, they could not analyze the depth of invasion independently from tumor stage. Despite this limitation, their study reveals that greater depth of invasion and higher tumor grade are correlated with increased angiogenesis. This suggests that angiogenic capacity may be one of the biological characteristics associated with endometrial tumor grade. The important message is that endometrial hyperplasia and endometrial carcinoma are angiogenic, and should therefore be detected by sensitive Doppler units. Furthermore, in stage I endometrial carcinoma, greater depth of invasion and higher tumor grade are directly correlated with angiogenic intensity.

Obviously, color and pulsed Doppler improve diagnostic accuracy, as most cases of endometrial carcinoma have abnormal blood flow (tumor angiogenesis)[14] with low impedance[15,16].

Bourne and colleagues[17] (Table 1) studied the impedance to blood flow in uterine arteries in patients with endometrial carcinoma and in those with normal endometrial morphology. They reported a significant difference in pulsatility index (PI) values between the groups and estimated the cut-off value of 2.00. In a subsequent publication[18], they reported an arbitrary cut-off value of 1.5 for uterine artery PI as a basis for a positive test result. It seems that the uterine artery itself is too large to show hemodynamic disturbances caused by small areas of neovascularization in the early stages of endometrial carcinoma. On the contrary, in the advanced stages, where specific vessels cannot be identified due to massive necrosis, uterine artery blood flow shows significant reduction in impedance. Hata and co-workers[19] (Table 1) measured the RI in the arcuate artery in patients with endometrial carcinoma. They found a significantly lower RI value (0.54 ± 0.16) compared to that of normal uteri ($RI = 0.77 \pm 0.75$). Merce and colleagues[20] studied 45 patients with metrorrhagia and compared their findings with 19 normal women. They measured the Doppler signals in both uterine arteries and within the myometrium, which they assumed to be in the vascular territory of the radial and arcuate arteries. A significant decrease in RI of the uterine and intramyometrial arteries was found in women with endometrial abnormalities, including two cases with endometrial carcinoma, compared with normal histology. The authors concluded that the RI of intramyometrial (arcuate and radial) arteries was highly accurate in predicting positive findings in comparison with the RI of uterine arteries, which was less accurate and less specific in predicting endometrial

Table 1 Blood flow characteristics in the detection of endometrial carcinoma

Reference	Number of patients with endometrial carcinoma	Uterine artery mean PI	Tumoral blood flow mean RI
Bourne et al.[17]	17	0.89	
Hata et al.[19]	10		0.54
Rudigoz and Gaucherand[21]	7		0.47–0.60
Kurjak et al.[23]	35		0.42
Ilijas et al.[24]	14		0.39
Allem et al.[25]	14		0.50

pathology. However, all the mentioned authors analyzed blood flow in pre-existing vessels (uterine, arcuate, or radial arteries).

Rudigoz and Gaucherand[21] (Table 1) proposed the combination of morphological (endometrial/uterine thickness ratio) and Doppler criteria for detection of endometrial malignancy. An abnormal blood flow pattern was found in six out of seven endometrial cancers with the RI ranging from 0.47 to 0.60.

Sladkevicius and associates[22] evaluated 138 women scheduled for curettage because of postmenstrual bleeding. They performed transvaginal ultrasound examination, including color and spectral Doppler analysis. They concluded that measurement of endometrial thickness with transvaginal ultrasonography is a better method for discriminating between benign and malignant or normal and pathological endometrium than is Doppler velocimetry of the uterine arteries.

However, there is an urgent need for standardization of Doppler measurements. Our group has proposed the following protocol.

B-mode imaging should be first used to evaluate:

(1) The endometrial thickness in longitudinal section, measured from the anterior subendometrial hypoechoic zone (halo) to the opposite side, thus including two endometrial layers;

(2) Echogenicity of the endometrium (hypoechogenic, hyperechogenic, or inhomogeneous) in relation to the endometrium;

(3) Presence or absence of the intracavitary fluid; and

(4) Integrity of the subendometrial (hypoechogenic) halo; when interrupted, the suspected depth of myometrial invasion was evaluated as being superficial (if infiltration was less than half of the myometrium) or deep (more than half).

Color Doppler should then be superimposed to evaluate:

(1) The presence or absence of vascular signals;

(2) The location of the tumoral blood vessels; described as intratumoral (within the endometrial echo);

(3) The measurement of the peak systolic velocities, and the impedance to blood flow (resistance index = RI). Women receiving hormonal replacement therapy (HRT) should have special attention as HRT is known to affect endometrial thickness and pelvic blood flow.

We will illustrate our own results obtained using the protocol described. A transvaginal color and pulsed Doppler study performed in our Department evaluated 750 postmenopausal women before hysterectomy for different gynecological indications[23] (Table 1). Of 750 women, 35 cases had endometrial carcinoma. Endometrial blood flow was absent in normal, atrophic and most cases of hyperplastic endometria; 91% of the cases of endometrial carcinoma displayed intratumoral and/or peritumoral blood flow (RI, 0.42 ± 0.02).

Of the endometrial carcinomas detected, 90% had an endometrial (tumoral) thickness of more than 10 mm (usually more than 20 mm); 10% of the endometrial carcinomas showed a thickness ranging from 5 to 10 mm. An endometrial thickness of less than 5 mm was consistent with 100% of atrophic and 73% of normal endometrium. Approximately half of the cases with endometrial carcinoma were presented either as hyperechoic or inhomogeneous. Although measurement of the endometrial thickness has been extensively studied, the importance of intrauterine fluid has received little attention. Its presence has been associated with malignancy of the genital tract, i.e. uterine, cervical, ovarian and tubal. The rule is that, once there is fluid in the uterus, a careful work-up for cancer detection is mandatory. In our study, the presence of significant intrauterine fluid in the uterus was consistent with endometrial carcinoma in most of the cases. However, absence of intracavitary fluid did not exclude malignancy. A subendometrial halo was visualized in 87% of detected endometrial carcinomas; the presence of an interrupted halo was consistent with myometrial invasion. The depth of myometrial invasion was evaluated as superficial (three cases) or deep (15 cases). The accuracy achieved in detecting myometrial invasion by sonography compared to histology was 92% with precise determination of its depth.

Areas of neovascularization were demonstrated in detected cases of endometrial carcinoma. The newly formed vessels were categorized as intratumoral (displaying colored zones within the endometrial echo) or peritumoral (displaying colored zones very close to the endometrial echo) (Figure 8). The intratumoral blood vessels displayed lower velocity than peritumoral blood vessels. The mean RI in tumoral blood vessels in cases with endometrial carcinoma was significantly lower than in those with endometrial hyperplasia (Figure 9). In this study, the features highly suggestive for endometrial carcinoma were:

(1) Endometrial thickness greater than 5 mm;

(2) Endometrial echoes inhomogeneous or hyperechoic; and

(3) Presence of intrauterine fluid.

Myometrial invasion was common when the subendometrial halo was interrupted. Intratumoral blood vessels displayed higher velocity than peritumoral blood vessels. A statistically significant difference was found between the mean RI in endometrial cancer and that in endometrial hyperplasia. This could have important clinical implications in differentiating between these entities *in vivo* (Table 2). Three cases were missed, as there was no endometrial tissue following dilatation and curettage operations performed within 1 week of scanning. This is an important observation which should be considered if optimal results are expected. Three cases with endometrial carcinoma stage I were

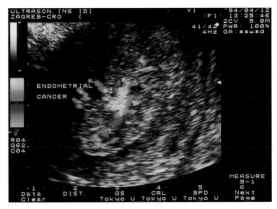

Figure 8 Thick inhomogeneous endometrium with star-like peripheral and intratumoral neovascularization seen by color flow imaging

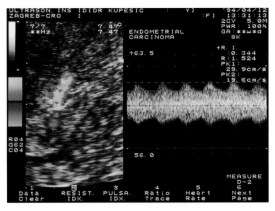

Figure 9 The same patient as in Figure 8. Pulsed Doppler waveform analysis (right) shows a low resistance index (RI = 0.34). Endometrial malignancy was confirmed by histopathology

Table 2 Blood flow visualization, resistance index, and peak systolic velocity in relation to histopathological characteristics

	n	Flow visualization rate		Resistance index		Peak systolic velocity	
		n	%	Mean	SD	Mean	SD
Atrophic	10	0	0	—	—	—	—
Normal	643	0	0	—	—	—	—
Hyperplastic	62	5	8	0.65*	0.05	7.2*	2.1
Endometrial carcinoma	35	32	91	0.42*	0.02	17.1*†	2.7

*$p < 0.05$; †peak systolic velocity detected only in peritumoral vessels

asymptomatic and discovered by the proposed protocol based on the presence of a thick endometrium (more than 20 mm) and intratumoral and/or peritumoral blood flow with a low RI.

In a more recent study from our Department, Ilijas and colleagues[24] (Table 1) analyzed 288 postmenopausal patients hysterectomized for different gynecological indications (incontinence, prolapse and descensus of uterus and myomas). Fourteen cases of endometrial carcinoma were diagnosed by histology. The detection rate of transvaginal color Doppler sonography in their study was 93%; out of 14 cases with endometrial carcinoma, 13 were detected by transvaginal color Doppler sonography. In 36% of patients with endometrial carcinoma, endometrial thickness was more than 10 mm; in 57% of patients endometrial thickness varied from 6 to 10 mm. In only one case with verified endometrial carcinoma, the endometrium measured 5 mm. Areas of neovascularization were demonstrated in 93% of patients with endometrial carcinoma. Newly formed vessels were categorized as intratumoral (displaying color-coded zones within the endometrial echo), and as peritumoral (displaying color-coded zones close to the echo pattern). The mean RI obtained from intratumoral blood vessels was 0.39 ± 0.03, and in peritumoral 0.43 ± 0.03. The RI values in cases with endometrial carcinoma had significantly lower values than in nine cases with endometrial hyperplasia with mean RI values 0.64 ± 0.05.

Allem and colleagues[25] (Table 1) tried to establish color and pulsed Doppler sonographic characteristics of uterine vascularity in postmenopausal patients with pathological endometrium in order to reduce the number of unnecessary diagnostic dilatation and curettage procedures. The prospective study involved 42 postmenopausal patients who were examined prior to the dilatation and curettage. Twenty patients had symptoms such as vaginal bleeding or clinically enlarged uterus and 22 postmenopausal women from their screening group were asymptomatic. Endometrial thickness (cut-off value of 8 mm), rates of visualization, and the density of uterine, myometrial (peritumoral) and endometrial (intratumoral) vessels were

used, along with the PI and RI of these vessels, to assess and correlate with endometrial pathology. Endometrial thickness was greater than 8 mm in all cases of endometrial carcinoma (14 of 14 cases), endometrial hyperplasia (eight of eight cases), and one endometrial polyp. In all cases of uterine myoma (nine cases) and in asymptomatic controls (11 subjects), the endometrial thickness was below 8 mm. The percentage of visualization of myometrial and endometrial vessels in cases of endometrial carcinoma was 93% and 43%, respectively, which was significantly higher than for cases with benign endometrium. A 'dense' vascular arrangement was found in approximately 80% of endometrial carcinoma cases, whereas a 'scattered' vascular arrangement was predominantly found in cases of endometrial hyperplasia. Endometrial or intratumoral vessels were found in 43% of endometrial carcinoma patients, whereas, in the case of endometrial hyperplasia, these vessels were demonstrated in only 12% of patients. Mean PI and RI values in endometrial vessels in cases of endometrial carcinoma were 0.73 ± 0.11 and 0.50 ± 0.05, respectively.

Hata and co-workers[26] examined the effectiveness of hypertensive intra-arterial chemotherapy for endometrial carcinoma using transvaginal color Doppler ultrasound and magnetic resonance imaging. The RI was obtained from intratumoral blood flow velocity waveforms by transvaginal color Doppler ultrasound and changes in RI were calculated. RI measurements did not correlate with tumor volume. A significant difference was noted between RI values before (mean = 0.58 ± 0.15) and after (mean = 0.77 ± 0.13) hypertensive intra-arterial chemotherapy. They concluded that transvaginal color Doppler is a pertinent diagnostic tool for precisely evaluating hemodynamic changes after hypertensive intra-arterial chemotherapy, reflecting the effect of this therapy in endometrial carcinoma.

To conclude, the application of transvaginal color Doppler to the general population for screening of endometrial carcinoma may be a viable option if combined with ovarian screening in the same scan. In this way, the capital costs would be shared, and an oncological preventive medicine for women could be created. The use of this technique could also result in a reduction in dilatation and curettage operations with considerable saving of both the potential risks and economic costs of the operation.

References

1. Kurjak, A., Kupesic, S., Zalud, I. and Predanic, M. (1995). Transvaginal color Doppler. In Dodson, M. G. (ed.) *Transvaginal Ultrasound*, pp. 325–39. (New York: Churchill Livingstone)
2. Fleischer, A. C., Kepple, D. M. and Entman, S. S. (1991). Transvaginal sonography of uterine disorders. In Timor-Tritsch, I. E. and Rottem, S. (eds.) *Transvaginal Sonography*, 2nd edn. (New York: Elsevier)
3. Du Bose, T. J., Hill, L. W. and Henningan, H. W. (1985). Sonography of arcuate uterine blood flow vessels. *J. Ultrasound Med.*, **4**, 229–33
4. Callen, P. W., De Martini, W. J. and Filly, R. A. (1979). The central uterine cavity echo: a useful sign on the ultrasonographic evaluation of the female pelvis. *Radiology*, **131**, 187–90
5. Bohlman, M. E., Ensor, R. E. and Sanders, R. C. (1987). Sonographic findings in adenomyosis of the uterus. *Am. J. Radiol.*, **148**, 765–6
6. Siedler, D., Lang, F. C., Jeffrey, R. B. and Wing, V. W. (1987). Uterine adenomyosis – a difficult sonographic diagnosis. *J. Ultrasound Med.*, **6**, 345–9
7. Soules, M. R. and McCarty, K. S. Jr (1982). Leiomyoma: steroid receptor content. Variation within normal menstrual cycles. *Am. J. Obstet. Gynecol.*, **143**, 6–11
8. Droegmueller, E. (1992). Endometriosis and adenomyosis. In Manning, S., Steinborn, E. and Salway, J. (eds.) *Comprehensive Gynecology*, pp. 545–76 (St Louis: Mosby Year Book)
9. Hirai, M., Shibata, K., Sagai, H., Sekiya, S. and Goldberg, B. B. (1995). Transvaginal pulsed and color Doppler sonography for the evaluation of adenomyosis. *J. Ultrasound Med.*, **14**, 529–32
10. Jurkovic, D., Bourne, T., Jauniaux, E., Campbell, S. and Collins, P. W. (1992). Transvaginal color Doppler study of blood flow in ectopic pregnancy. *Fertil. Steril.*, **57**, 68–73
11. Stabile, I., Grudzinskas, J. and Campbell, S. (1990). Doppler ultrasonographic evaluation of abnormal pregnancies in the first trimester. *J. Clin. Ultrasound*, **18**, 497–501
12. Jauniaux, E., Jurkovic, D. and Campbell, S. (1991). *In vivo* investigation of the anatomy and the physiology of early human placental circulations. *Ultrasound Obstet. Gynecol.*, **1**, 435–45
13. Abulafia, O., Triest, W. E., Sherer, D. M., Hansen, C. C. and Ghezzi, F. (1995). Angiogenesis in endometrial hyperplasia and stage I endometrial carcinoma. *Obstet. Gynecol.*, **86**, 479–85
14. Folkman, J., Cole, D. and Becker, F. (1963). Growth and metastasis of tumor in organ culture. *Tumor Res.*, **16**, 453–67
15. Kurjak, A. and Kupesic, S. (1995). Transvaginal color Doppler and pelvic tumor vascularity: lessons learned and future challenges. *Ultrasound Obstet. Gynecol.*, **6**, 1–15
16. Kurjak, A., Shalan, S., Kupesic, S., Predanic, I., Zalud, I., Breyer, B. and Jukic, S. (1993). Transvaginal color Doppler sonography in the assessment of pelvic tumor vascularity. *Ultrasound Obstet. Gynecol.*, **3**, 137–54
17. Bourne, T. H., Campbell, S., Whitehead, M. I., Royston, P., Steer, C. V. and Collins, W. P. (1990). Detection of endometrial cancer in postmenopausal women by transvaginal ultrasonography and color flow imaging. *Br. Med. J.*, **310**, 369–70
18. Bourne, T. H., Campbell, S., Steer, C. V., Royston, P., Whitehead, M. I. and Collins, W. P. (1991). Detection of endometrial cancer by transvaginal ultrasonography with color flow imaging and blood flow analysis: a preliminary report. *Gynecol. Oncol.*, **40**, 253–9
19. Hata, K., Makihara, K. and Hata, T. (1991). Transvaginal color Doppler imaging for hemodynamic assessment of reproductive tract tumors. *Jpn. Int. J. Gynecol. Obstet.*, **36**, 301–8
20. Merce, L. T., Garcia, L. and De La Fuente, F. (1991). Doppler ultrasound assessment of endometrial pathology. *Acta Obstet. Scand.*, **70**, 525–30
21. Rudigoz, R. C. and Gaucherand, P. (1993). Vaginal sonography and color Doppler in postmenopausal patients. *Ultrasound Obstet. Gynecol.*, **3**(Suppl. 2), 42
22. Sladkevicius, P., Valentin, L. and Marsal, K. (1994). Endometrial thickness and Doppler velocimetry of the uterine arteries as discriminators of endometrial status in women with postmenopausal bleeding: a comparative study. *Am. J. Obstet. Gynecol.*, **171**, 722–8
23. Kurjak, A., Shalan, H., Sosic, A., Benic, S., Zudenigo, D., Kupesic, S. and Predanic, M.

(1993). Endometrial carcinoma in post-menopausal women: evaluation by transvaginal color Doppler ultrasonography. *Am. J. Obstet. Gynecol.*, **169**, 1597–603

24. Ilijas, M., Marton, U. and Hanzevacki, M. (1996). Color Doppler in the assessment of endometrial carcinoma. In Kurjak, A. and Kupesic, S. (eds.) *Doppler in Gynecology and Infertility*, pp. 134–7. (Rome: Edizioni Internazionali)

25. Alleem, F., Predanic, M., Calame, R., Moukhtar, M. and Pennisi, J. (1995). Transvaginal color and pulsed Doppler sonography of the endometrium: a possible role in reducing the number of dilatation and curettage procedures. *J. Ultrasound Med.*, **14**, 139–45

26. Hata, K., Hata, T., Fujiwaki, R., Manabe, A. and Kitao, M. (1995). Hypertensive intra-arterial chemotherapy for endometrial carcinoma assessed by transvaginal Doppler ultrasound and magnetic resonance imaging. *J. Clin. Ultrasound*, **23**, 407–11

Effect of hormone replacement therapy on uterine blood flow and endometrial status in postmenopausal women

10

F. Bonilla-Musoles and M. C. Marti

INTRODUCTION

The life expectancy of women in developed countries has increased from 40 years at the beginning of the twentieth century to the current life expectancy of 85 years. Modern women spend one-third of their lives in a hormone-deficient state. The effect of hormone replacement therapy (HRT) on uterine vascular flow and endometrial thickness deserves special attention[1].

The fluximetric indices, detected by color Doppler, as well as the ultrasound image and the endometrial thickness, are different in women of reproductive age than in postmenopausal women[2,3].

It is important to understand the vascular effects of HRT and the effects on the postmenopausal endometrium for several reasons. An increasing number of menopausal women are on HRT. It is essential to distinguish physiological from pathological changes in these women. The physician must be able to recognize the HRT-induced thickened endometrium, considered pathological in the untreated postmenopausal woman.

The epidemiological data indicate that HRT has a protective effect on coronary artery disease in postmenopausal women, but the mechanism by which HRT influences arterial tone remains uncertain. It has been proposed that HRT has direct effects on arterial tone, called the 'nonmetabolic or direct vascular effects'[4].

Transvaginal color Doppler sonography (TVDS) is a relatively new technique that permits non-invasive evaluation of uterine hemodynamic status[2,5,6].

The advent of color imaging has significantly facilitated identification of vessels, and pulsatility index (PI) and resistance index (RI) are now considered the measurements of choice that represent the vessel distal tone[7].

Although there is some evidence that estrogens influence arterial tone[8-10], the vascular effects of HRT have not been fully defined. Furthermore, some of the studies have addressed the question of the combined estrogen–progestogen therapy[10]. The influence of the gestagenic addition on the beneficial direct vascular effects of HRT has not yet been determined in the human. Moreover, there is a lack of studies comparing sequential and continuous gestagenic addition regimens.

Preliminary reports[11] indicate that HRT remains effective during several months of treatment, but the impact of long-term hormonal use is unknown.

Although HRT is widely used in postmenopausal women, questions still remain regarding its safety and mode of action. There is evidence that endometrial thickness changes with HRT[5,12-14], but new sonographic criteria are needed for postmenopausal women receiving HRT, in order to establish optimal management protocols and replacement guidelines.

We are going to comment here on most of the studies of HRT effects, reporting also our own results on this issue[15–17]. A total of 345 women who were at least 1 year postmenopausal and who had unremarkable obstetric and gynecological histories gave informed consent to participate in our study on the vascular and endometrial effects of HRT. At each visit, we performed an ultrasound assessment of the uterus (including endometrial thickness) and of the blood flow in the uterine arteries, measuring PI and RI. All women were screened for abnormal masses, uterine myomata and endometrial polyps during ultrasound examinations.

The mean age of the women studied was 52.1 years, with a range of 39–70 (four patients with proved premature menopause were included, and their age range was 28–35 years). The mean time since menopause of the women studied was 4.3 years (range 1–20), the median being 2.5 years.

Of these women, 247 reported no history of HRT. Ninety-eight women were already on an HRT program when the study was started. One hundred and forty-two women opted not to begin an HRT regimen after the initial TVDS evaluation. One hundred and five women who had never been on HRT elected to start on one of the regimens we offered following the initial TVDS evaluation. Because after 1 year no statistically significant differences were seen between women who began HRT in our study and those who were already on treatment when they entered it, all treated women were placed in one of the three groups according to the HRT regimen they were following.

(1) Group 1: 58 women on ERT (unopposed estrogen therapy). These women were treated with continuous transdermal 17β-estradiol (17β-E$_2$) (0.05 mg/day, Estraderm TTS, Ciba-Geigy, Summit, NJ).

(2) Group 2: 85 women were on combined continuous HRT. These women were treated with continuous transdermal estradiol (as described) and 2.5 mg/day (30 women) or 5 mg/day (35 women) of medroxyprogesterone acetate (Progevera, Upjohn, Kalamazoo, MI) was added continuously. In 20 women, we added 100 mg/day of natural progesterone.

(3) Group 3: 60 women were given combined sequential HRT. The progestogen added to the continuous estradiol was, in 30 women, 10 mg/day of medroxyprogesterone acetate; and in 30 women 200 mg/day of natural progesterone. The progestogen was added from day 17 to day 28 of each 28-day cycle.

Patients on HRT had an examination prior to treatment. After that, they had repeated TVDS examinations, the first on day 26 of the first cycle, and then every 3 months during the 1 year of therapy. We excluded the assessments after 1 year, because not all the patients had completed more than 12 months on HRT. Women in the third group had their first post-treatment examination on day 13 and the second on day 26 of the first cycle.

Twelve women who had baseline studies prior to beginning HRT had TVDS examinations weekly during the 1st month of therapy. Four of these women were on an unopposed ERT regimen. Four women were on a continuous combined estrogen–progestogen regimen, and four of them were on the combined sequential estrogen–progestogen regimen. Linear regression analysis, analysis of variance (ANOVA), and paired and unpaired Student's t-test, where appropriate, were used for statistical analysis. A 99% or a 95% confidence interval was selected.

The object of our study was to determine whether HRT had a direct effect on uterine arterial blood flow. If there is an effect, we wanted to establish whether it occurs shortly after the onset of therapy, and whether it changes with time (long-term effects of HRT). We also wished to know whether the addition of a progestogen altered the vascular response to estrogen therapy, also comparing the sequential and the continuous combined HRT regimens.

NORMAL UTERINE ARTERY BLOOD FLOW IN POSTMENOPAUSAL WOMEN

It is necessary to establish normal fluximetric reference values in postmenopausal women, in order to assess the effects that HRT administration has on uterine and endometrial blood flow indices, and also to select more efficiently women who are at risk for uterine malignancy.

Referring to blood flow indices in uterine arteries, it is unusual to find a PI below 3.0 and a RI below 0.9[5,12,18,19]. According to these data, the vascular map we obtained in the 345 postmenopausal women assessed was represented by a PI mean value of 3.38 ± 0.98 and a RI mean value of 0.92 ± 0.09, meaning that vascular resistance increases at the menopause, compared with the women's fertile age[1,12]. No correlation was found between the PI and RI values and the age of the women.

We found that uterine arterial PI and RI values were correlated with time since menopause, that is, the longer the time since menopause, the higher the RI and PI values. This significant positive correlation between uterine vascular impedance to flow and number of years since menopause, was found for both PI ($p < 0.0001$) and RI ($p < 0.0001$). Figures 1 and 2 show the relationship of RI (Figure 1) and PI (Figure 2) with time since menopause.

A subgroup of women was found to have PI values below 3 and RI values below 0.9. Analyzing their medical histories, we found two variables that seemed to modify the indices values.

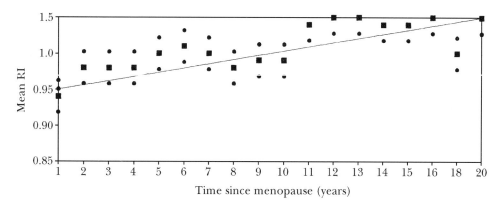

Figure 1 Relationship of resistance index (RI) with time since menopause. Linear regression and statistical analysis were performed with all the RI values, although only mean values (squares) with SEM (dots) are represented in order to get an easier visual effect; $p < 0.0001$, $r = 0.31$

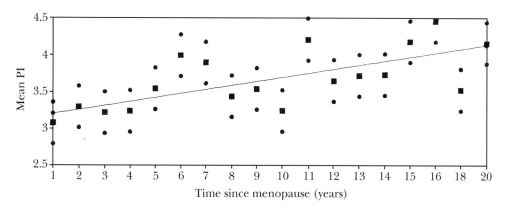

Figure 2 Relationship of pulsatility index (PI) with time since menopause. Linear regression and statistical analysis were performed with all the PI values, although only mean values (squares) with SEM (dots) are represented in order to get an easier visual effect; $p < 0.0001$, $r = 0.29$

First, there were 23 postmenopausal women who were taking medications known to have vascular effects. Among drugs that may influence arterial blood flow are cardioactive, psychotropic, anti-varicose and anti-hypertensive medications. This group of patients had significantly lower ($p < 0.0001$) (Figure 3) RI and PI ($p < 0.0001$) values than the rest of the postmenopausal women who were not taking such medications. Also, there was another group of 15 women in which we detected the presence of remaining vascular ovarian activity (detectable ovarian artery flow), that disappeared spontaneously on subsequent examinations. In 13 of these women the time since menopause was 1 year; one woman was 3 years and another was 4 years postmenopausal. These women had significantly lower values of RI ($p < 0.0001$) and PI ($p < 0.001$) indices, as shown in Figure 4 for the PI.

Nevertheless, in both subgroups (women taking vasoactive medications, and women with remaining vascular ovarian activity) with lower indices values, the PI and RI values were also higher as the time since menopause increased.

So, if we aim to establish reference value parameters of uterine blood flow indices in postmenopausal women, the most interesting parameter to take into account is the elapsed time since menopause. As preliminary reports indicate[8,10], and according to our current results[15], there is a relationship of both fluximetric blood flow indices (PI and RI) with time since menopause.

Gangar and co-workers[9] found that there was a correlation between PI values and time since

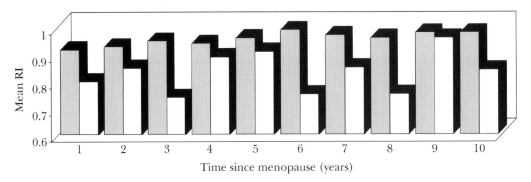

Figure 3 Resistance index values in populations with (hollow columns) and without (grey columns) vasoactive medication at the different times since menopause studied. Time-matched values between groups were compared using analysis of variance (ANOVA); $p < 0.0001$, $r = 0.49$

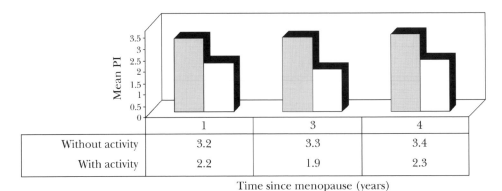

	1	3	4
Without activity	3.2	3.3	3.4
With activity	2.2	1.9	2.3

Time since menopause (years)

Figure 4 Pulsatility index values in women with (hollow columns) and without (gray columns) remaining vascular ovarian activity at the different times since menopause studied. Numerical mean values are given in table below. Time-matched values between groups were compared using analysis of variance (ANOVA)

menopause, after studying blood flow in the internal carotid arteries of ten postmenopausal women. Hillard and colleagues[10] found the same relationship between PI in uterine arteries and time since menopause, in the pretreatment assessment of their 2-month study of HRT effects on 12 postmenopausal women. In contrast to these authors, and also to our results, Zalud and colleagues[14] assessed the RI values on 109 menopausal women, finding that, even though RI values were higher as the time since menopause increased, this relationship does not reach statistical significance, but, as the authors state in their work, left and right RI values in individual patients were poorly correlated at each assessment, and thus they presented the results for both arteries separately.

Our results[15], that confirm the previous observations of others[9,10] show that there is a poor relationship of both PI ($p < 0.0001$, $r = 0.29$) and RI ($p < 0.0001$, $r = 0.31$) with time since menopause. Both PI and RI values slowly increase as time since menopause increases. This relationship has a high statistical significance ($p < 0.0001$). Nevertheless, the fact that a person's correlation of the linear regression is not so high can be explained in terms of other parameters (psychosocial, dietary and health factors)[4] that are also determining local and/or systemic blood flow.

EFFECTS OF HORMONE REPLACEMENT ON UTERINE BLOOD FLOW IN POST-MENOPAUSAL WOMEN

Pulsatility and resistance indices are indicators of resistance to flow distal to the point of measurement. The higher the value, the greater the resistance and vice versa.

After the pretreatment assessment, and once HRT was administered, we measured PI and RI in uterine arteries, finding that HRT lowered both indices; they went from a mean PI of 3.38 ± 0.98 and a mean RI of 0.92 ± 0.09 in the pretreatment, to a PI mean value of 2.00 ± 0.55 and a mean RI of 0.79 ± 0.08 at the first HRT assessment, on day 26 of the first HRT cycle.

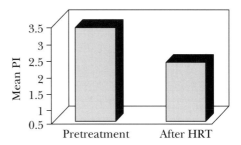

Figure 5 Pulsatility index (PI) values after HRT: the effects observed before HRT and in the first assessment. The median fall in PI was 35% ($p < 0.0001$)

In the first cycle, the mean PI fell to 65 ± 19% ($p < 0.0001$) and the RI fell to 87 ± 7% ($p < 0.0001$) of their pretreatment values, at the first on-treatment assessment, on day 26 (Figure 5).

In the group on sequential gestagenic addition, measurements were performed on day 13 and day 26 of the cycle. No statistical differences in PI and RI values between unopposed estrogen therapy and combined (estrogen–progestogen) hormone replacement were found, nor were any found between continuous and sequential gestagenic addition groups.

As there were no differences with any of the three regimens of therapy, the data of the three groups have been combined. The results from the three regimens are shown in Tables 1 and 2.

In order to clarify HRT effects on this first on-treatment cycle, we assessed 12 of our patients weekly during their first HRT cycle. Again, we found no differences in PI and RI values depending on the regimen of therapy administered. At the 1st week assessment, we found that the significant fall in PI and RI values had already taken place. The lowered PI and RI values remained so in the 2nd, 3rd and 4th week (day 26) assessments. These results are presented in Figure 6, and the table below presents the mean value at each assessment.

It has already been reported[9,10,15] that there is a significant correlation of PI and RI values with time since menopause, in untreated postmenopausal women. Statistically significant correlation between HRT effect (lowering of PI and RI values from pretreatment to the first on-treatment assessment) and time since menopause

($p < 0.0001$) was only found for PI. The longer the time since menopause, the greater the fall in PI and RI values (Figure 7).

When comparing the progestogens used in combined HRT, no significant differences were found between medroxyprogesterone acetate,

Table 1 Changes in pulsatility index following HRT administration (means ± SD)

	Pretreatment	1st cycle on HRT (day 26)	Change (%)
HRT	3.38 ± 0.98	2.00 ± 0.55	35 ± 19
Unopposed ERT	3.35 ± 0.91	1.86 ± 0.47	36 ± 17
Combined HRT	3.39 ± 1.15	2.06 ± 0.58	35 ± 20
continuous HRT	3.65 ± 1.26	2.16 ± 0.69	38 ± 22
sequential HRT	3.16 ± 0.79	1.97 ± 0.44	32 ± 18

Table 2 Changes in resistance index following HRT administration (means ± SD)

	Pretreatment	1st cycle on HRT (day 26)	Change (%)
HRT	0.92 ± 0.09	0.79 ± 0.08	13 ± 7
Unopposed ERT	0.94 ± 0.09	0.78 ± 0.08	13 ± 8
Combined HRT	0.91 ± 0.11	0.80 ± 0.08	12.5 ± 9
continuous HRT	0.91 ± 0.12	0.81 ± 0.08	13 ± 7
sequential HRT	0.91 ± 0.08	0.79 ± 0.08	12 ± 9

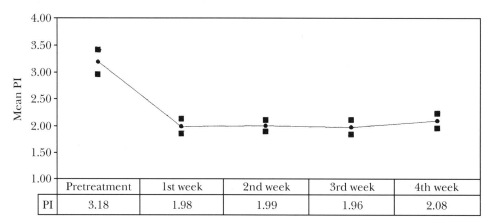

Figure 6 Pulsatility index (PI) values at the weekly follow-up in the first treatment cycle. Solid squares indicate confidence intervals

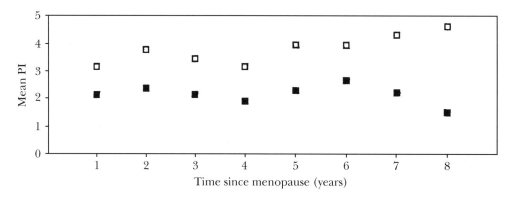

Figure 7 Variation in pulsatility index (PI) after HRT in relation to years after the menopause. Open squares, pretreatment; solid squares, on HRT; $p < 0.05$, $r = 0.29$

that resulted in a mean PI of 2.17 ± 0.67 and a mean RI of 0.81 ± 0.09, and natural progesterone, with a PI mean value of 2.23 ± 0.88 and a RI mean value of 0.83 ± 0.10 ($p < 0.05$; paired t-test).

Hormone replacement therapy and cardiovascular disease

There has been uncertainty, and even controversy, addressing the question whether HRT reduces the risk of cardiovascular disease in postmenopausal women. This issue has been recently reviewed, and the most extensive analysis[20,21] indicates a 40–50% reduction in risk of coronary artery disease attributable to estrogen replacement.

Because arterial disease is the most common cause of death in women over 50 years in industrialized countries, this protective effect of ERT (estrogen replacement therapy) has major health implications. Postmenopausal hormone therapy is now considered as a legitimate component of preventive health care for older women.

Most of the epidemiological evidence indicates that estrogen replacement therapy reduces the risk of coronary artery disease[21], but how this protection is mediated remains uncertain. Since less than 50% of this protection is mediated by the beneficial effects due to lipid metabolism[22], it was proposed that HRT has direct effects on arterial tone. These effects have been called 'non-metabolic or direct vascular effects'[4].

Estrogens exert many direct effects on the cardiovascular system that are independent of the metabolic changes. There are a limited number of markers of these direct arterial effects. Currently, only the vascular response to acetylcholine, and the PI and the RI reflecting changes in blood flow, are viewed as useful markers.

Our current results[16] confirm previous observations of others[10,19] that both the PI and the RI of the uterine arteries are reduced as an immediate effect of HRT administration. This effect is profound, with a significant reduction in mean PI of 35% ($p < 0.0001$), and of 13% in mean RI ($p < 0.0001$). We found that the decrease in PI and RI had already taken place at the 1st-week assessment. After the 1st week, PI and RI values remained the same.

The vascular response induced by HRT is also quick, because it has already taken place within 7 days of HRT administration. This means that whatever the mechanism, HRT acts quickly. There is an increase in pelvic arterial flow mapping following HRT. Uterine arterial RI and PI are significantly decreased in women undergoing HRT. The only contrary report of this vascular response has been made by Zalud and co-workers[14]. They investigated the changes in endometrial and myometrial thickness in 109 women, 20 of whom were on HRT. They studied the vascular blood changes. Surprisingly, the RI did not vary with HRT administration, nor with time since menopause. This observation differs from all other published reports and may reflect a different response to patch vs. oral administration.

Nevertheless, we have already assessed[15,16] that individual blood flow in uterine arteries of postmenopausal women is correlated with several variables. Because the pretreatment PI and RI were related to time since menopause, we investigated if the response to treatment (lowering of both indices from pretreatment to first HRT assessment) was also related to time since menopause, finding that this correlation was significant only for the PI ($p < 0.05$). With these current results, we cannot be certain that the longer the time since menopause, the greater the response to HRT. What we can be sure of is that the vascular response to HRT was found equally despite the length of time since menopause, perhaps even greater. This would have an important impact on clinical outcome, for it means that older women with a long time since menopause will enjoy the protective vascular effects of HRT.

It has been assessed that there is a vascular response to HRT. As had been reported[10], if these described changes in arterial tone are one of the important mechanisms by which HRT reduces arterial disease risk, then it would be predictable that the cardiovascular benefits will be of rapid onset, and will also be observed in women that have started HRT a long time after the menopause.

HRT vascular effect as a generalized phenomenon

It might be argued that the profound response of uterine arteries to HRT could occur only in the pelvic vasculature, which could be particularly susceptible to gonadal hormones. However, similar investigations that have assessed blood flow in other human vessels suggest we are before a generalized phenomenon. Several authors have found, in the internal carotid artery[9], and in the middle cerebral arteries[23], a significant decrease in PI after HRT administration, assessed at weeks 6[23] or 9[9] on HRT. With Doppler echocardiography[11], a significant increase has been found in all parameters of blood flow in the aorta of 24 women on HRT.

The results that we[16,17], and also others[10,14,19,24] report from uterine arteries, together with other human vessels, show that the important decrease in PI and RI after HRT administration can be now considered as the consequence of a generalized reactivity (maybe locally different) of arteries to estradiol in all human vessels. This HRT effect on vascular reactivity increases peripheral blood flow and can be considered as one of the mechanisms by which estrogens have a protective effect against coronary artery disease.

Long-term HRT effects

Investigations studying combined HRT vascular effects have been made with a limited number of patients, and on a very short term (from two cycles, up to a maximum of 6 months). So, there is a lack of studies addressing the long-term effects of combined HRT. Preliminary reports[11,18] indicate that HRT vascular effects remain the same after at least 6 months of use.

We have performed examinations after the first HRT cycle, and then every 3 months during 12 months of treatment. We found that, after the fall detected at the 1st week of therapy, PI and RI values remained almost the same through all the 12 months assessed. The differences between all assessments were not statistically significant (analysis of variance, $p > 0.05$) (Figure 8). With these results, according with those found in other vessels[11], we can conclude that HRT maintains all its beneficial vascular effects, at least during the 1 year on therapy assessed.

Vascular effects of combined HRT regimens

The need for a combined estrogen–progestogen regimen in postmenopausal hormone

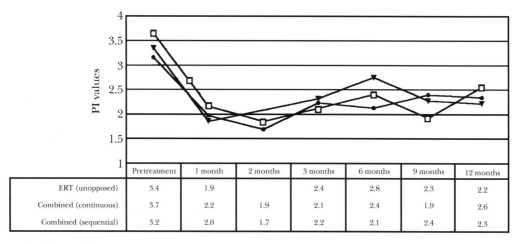

	Pretreatment	1 month	2 months	3 months	6 months	9 months	12 months
ERT (unopposed)	3.4	1.9		2.4	2.8	2.3	2.2
Combined (continuous)	3.7	2.2	1.9	2.1	2.4	1.9	2.6
Combined (sequential)	3.2	2.0	1.7	2.2	2.1	2.4	2.3

Figure 8 The evolution of the pulsatility index (PI) in relation to time of HRT therapy. Solid triangles, unopposed ERT; open squares, combined (continuous) HRT; solid circles, combined (sequential) HRT

replacement to prevent endometrial carcinoma is accepted worldwide. There are many reports about the effects of gestagenic addition on lipid metabolism[25]. Several metabolic parameters seem to be less favorably affected when combined therapy is prescribed; results are not conclusive[26], because the combination metabolic effects are dependent on the route of administration of the estrogen, the type of progestogen and the dosages.

Even more uncertainty remains as to whether the addition of progestogen would have any antagonistic effect on the described protective 'direct vascular effect' of estrogens in coronary artery disease risk. In animal investigations, it has been demonstrated that the addition of progesterone had no effect on the beneficial effect seen in the unopposed ERT group. Both groups showed significantly less atherogenesis (the combined group showed even less atherogenesis than the unopposed estrogens group). In the human, although there are some studies that have addressed this question[18,24], the influence of the gestagenic addition over the beneficial direct vascular effects of HRT has not yet been determined.

Hillard and co-workers[10] studied the vascular effect of gestagenic addition in the uterine arteries of 11 postmenopausal women, and they conclude that, if there is any adverse effect due to progestogens on the estrogen-induced change, it is partial and of short duration.

We compared 59 women on ERT with 137 women on combined HRT (with gestagenic addition). We found no statistical differences in PI and RI values between unopposed estrogen therapy and combined (estrogen–progestogen) hormone replacement, as shown in Tables 1 and 2.

Our current results[16], according with previous observations of others[23,24], confirm there is no effect due to the addition of progestogens on the estradiol-mediated vascular response that has been assessed.

Referring to the investigation of the effects of combined HRT regimens, there is a lack of comparative studies between sequential and continuous regimens of progestogen addition. In our study, we found no significant differences

between continuous and sequential gestagenic addition groups. We analyzed also if there were any changes in HRT effects depending on the gestagen used in combined HRT. No significant differences were found between medroxyprogesterone acetate and natural progesterone.

Thus, the assessment of an absence of adverse effects due to the addition of progesterone on the estradiol-mediated vascular response has important clinical implications, as it means that the protective cardiovascular effect attributed to estrogens is also observed when combined HRT regimens are administered.

ENDOMETRIAL STATUS: EFFECTS OF HORMONE REPLACEMENT ON POSTMENOPAUSAL WOMEN

After the assessment of endometrial status in postmenopausal women, no relationship of endometrial thickness with time since menopause was found.

Endometrial thickness measurement in postmenopausal women before HRT (baseline) resulted in a mean value of 2.52 ± 2.65 mm (range 0–16 mm), and, once HRT was administered, the endometrial thickness increased up to a mean of 4.92 ± 3.73 mm (range 0–19 mm).

An increase in endometrial thickness was evident soon after HRT administration. HRT induced a highly significant thickening of the endometrial line ($p < 0.0001$), as represented in Figure 9. Depending on the regimen of therapy employed, the HRT-induced thickening of the endometrium differs, the differences between the three (types of therapy) regimens being statistically significant ($p < 0.05$). The sequential

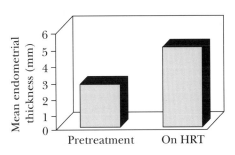

Figure 9 Endometrial thickness modification after HRT

addition of gestagen provoked the maximum thickening of the endometrial line, while the slightest one was due to the continuous gestagen path, giving the greatest difference between these two regimens ($p < 0.0001$).

From 345 asymptomatic postmenopausal women studied, we found an endometrial line > 5 mm in 21 cases (8%). On proceeding to endometrial sampling and histopathological study, we found the majority had an atrophic endometrium. From 287 postmenopausal women receiving HRT, an endometrial line > 5 mm was found in 94 women (33% of cases). In these 94 women with an endometrial line > 5 mm, the histopathological study demonstrated mainly proliferative changes (62%).

HRT induced a significant increase in the number of women whose endometrial line was > 5 mm ($p < 0.0001$), this percentage being statistically different in the three regimens of treatment ($p < 0.001$), for we found 22% in the unopposed estrogen group, 35% in the sequential gestagen group, and finally, only 15% in the continuous gestagenic addition group. These results are presented in Figure 10, where we can see the main differences are between the continuous and sequential gestagenic addition.

The histopathological changes induced by HRT (in women with an endometrial line > 5 mm) are presented in Figure 11. No differences between the three regimens were found.

Endometrial thickness mean values found in each histopathological type are presented in Table 3. Endometrial thicknesses are different depending on the histological basis, although they only reach statistical significance if we consider atrophic and proliferative endometrium on the one side, and hyperplasia and adenocarcinoma on the other ($p < 0.0001$). Results from the histological samples of women with an endometrial line > 5 mm (21/243 in women without prior therapy and 81/298 in the treated group) demonstrated endometrial hyperplasia or adenocarcinoma only in women whose endometrial line was greater than 9 mm (Figure 12). All other women had only proliferative endometrium with a normal appearance.

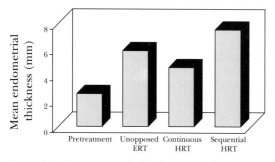

Figure 10 Endometrial thickness modifications after HRT according to the type of therapy used

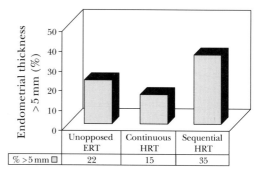

Figure 11 Number of patients with endometrial thickness > 5 mm according to the type of therapy used

Table 3 Endometrial thickness mean values in women with endometrial line (EL) > 5 mm for each histopathological type

	Non-treated		On HRT	
	Mean endometrial thickness (mm)	Cases with EL > 5 mm (%)	Mean endometrial thickness (mm)	Cases with EL > 5 mm (%)
Atrophic endometrium	8.1	47.6	8.3	24.7
Proliferative endometrium	9.4	38.1	8.4	61.8
Hyperplasia	11.0	9.5	13.7	12.3
Endometrial carcinoma	16.0	4.8	19.0	1.2

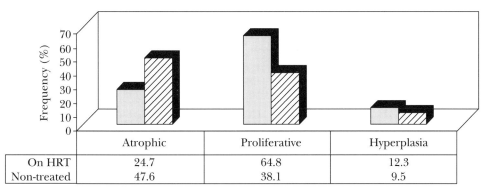

	Atrophic	Proliferative	Hyperplasia
On HRT	24.7	64.8	12.3
Non-treated	47.6	38.1	9.5

Figure 12 The frequencies of different histopathological findings in patients with endometrial thickness > 5 mm. Gray columns, on HRT; hatched columns, non-treated

No relationship between the presence of metrorrhagia with endometrial thickness was found, nor was it a determining parameter in the resulting histology.

In women receiving HRT, we also investigated the presence of intraendometrial flow, finding it appeared in two cases of proliferative endometrium (3.6%), in five women with hyperplasia (45.5%) and in the women with carcinoma (100%).

We had two cases of carcinoma, one in an asymptomatic postmenopausal woman detected in the baseline assessment, and the other in the first assessment of a nurse taking HRT without medical control. In both cases, we found intraendometrial flow (mean RI = 0.42; PI = 0.50), and both uterine artery indices were very low (mean RI = 0.69; PI = 1.1), the differences with either postmenopausal untreated women (mean PI = 3.38 ± 0.98; mean RI = 0.92 ± 0.09) or even with women receiving HRT (mean PI = 2.0 ± 0.55; mean RI = 0.79 ± 0.08) being highly significant ($p < 0.001$).

The earliest reports about changes in endometrial thickness with the effect of different dosages of estrogen and progesterone indicated a thickening of the endometrial line greater than 5 mm (the established limit for menopausal women) in more than 50% of cases. Zalud and colleagues[14] investigated the changes in endometrial and myometrial thickness in 109 women, 20 of whom were on HRT. Women on HRT had an endometrial thickness greater than 5 mm, regardless of age. The average thickness

Table 4 HRT effects on endometrial thickness (EL)

	Non-treated	On HRT
Mean EL (mm)	2.52	4.92
Cases with EL > 5 mm (%)	8	33
unopposed ERT	—	22
continuous HRT	—	15
sequential HRT	—	35

was 7.7 mm. Our current results[17] indicate that HRT induces a highly significant thickening of the endometrial line ($p < 0.0001$), that differs depending on the regimen of therapy employed, the differences between the three types of therapy being statistically significant ($p < 0.05$). The sequential addition of gestagen provoked the maximum thickening of the endometrial line, while the slightest one was due to the continuous gestagen path, meeting the greatest difference between these two regimens ($p < 0.0001$).

Endometrial thickness measurement has been introduced as a routine procedure for the screening of endometrial carcinoma. It has been suggested[27] that an endometrial thickness of 5 mm is an appropriate cut-off level for conservative management of patients with postmenopausal bleeding or in screening for endometrial carcinoma. Endometrial measurement has high sensitivity but very low specificity in screening for endometrial carcinoma. In addition, HRT increases endometrial thickness significantly especially the sequential addition of the gestagen regimen. For all these reasons, it results in ambiguous findings when endometrial thickness measurement is undertaken for screening malignancy.

The acknowledgement of the HRT-induced endometrial changes is of major importance in clinical practice, for it is important to be able to distinguish physiological situations from pathological endometrial changes in postmenopausal women. Furthermore, it should be taken into account that the thickened endometrium induced by HRT is considered a 'physiological' change dependent upon the patient's hormonal status[1].

The main diagnostic trouble is that we, and other authors[17], found an overlap in endometrial thickness between those women with endometrial malignancy and those without. In addition to this, the diagnosis becomes more difficult, for the overlap is greater, in women taking HRT, due to the 'physiological' hormone-induced thickened endometrium that these women have.

Endometrial carcinoma is the cause of postmenopausal bleeding in only 10% of cases[28]. It has been shown that these malignant tumors are associated with neoangiogenesis[29]. Bourne and co-workers[12] reported the presence of small low-resistance vessels in postmenopausal women with endometrial cancer. Our results, however, suggest that low-resistance vessels may also occur in other conditions. We detected them in one patient who had endometrial hyperplasia, one with an endometrial polyp, and following HRT in two patients with submucous myomata.

In our cases of endometrial cancer[17], agreeing with other authors[13], the tumors showed signs of altered vascularization, presenting endometrial flow with very low resistance ($RI = 0.42$; $PI = 0.50$) and also showed a statistically significant lower PI and RI in uterine arteries ($p < 0.0001$) compared with the rest of postmenopausal women (including women receiving HRT).

Finally, we believe, according to others[13,14], that in the screening for endometrial carcinoma on postmenopausal women it is essential to take into account the 'physiologic' hormone-dependent endometrial thickening of the women receiving HRT. We believe there is a need to establish new cut-off levels (for conservative management of patients) that allow for changes in endometrial thickness during HRT.

CONCLUSIONS

In summary, vascular resistance in uterine arteries increases at the menopause and becomes higher as time since menopause increases.

Nevertheless, there are other variables that should be taken into account. The eventual detection of remaining vascular ovarian activity and some vasoactive medications lower the values of both indices. Other variables (e.g. dietary and psychosocial factors) that determine systemic blood flow can also determine local uterine blood flow in postmenopausal women and should be considered.

Postmenopausal women have a rapid and profound uterine vascular flow response to HRT. If these described changes in arterial tone are one of the important mechanisms by which HRT reduces arterial disease risk, then there is no effect due to the addition of progesterone on the estradiol-mediated vascular response that has been assessed. HRT maintains all its beneficial vascular effects, at least during the 1 year of therapy assessed. It is predictable that the cardiovascular benefits will be of rapid onset, and will also be observed in women that have started HRT a long time after the menopause.

Referring to endometrial status, transvaginal Doppler sonography, especially with color flow imaging to assess uterine artery blood flow characteristics, can be useful to detect endometrial carcinoma in postmenopausal women. The screening procedure must take into account endometrial and uterine blood flow changes that occur when menopausal women are on HRT.

References

1. Lin, M. C., Goskink, B. B., Wolf, S. I., Fedesmaln, M. R., Stuenkel, C. A., Braly, P. S., and Pretorius, D. H. (1991). Endometrial thickness after menopause: effect of hormone replacement. *Radiology*, **180**(2), 427–32

2. Crvencovic, G., Karlon, B. Y., Smart, C. L., Cane, P., Sarti, D. A. and Platt, L. D. (1992). Transvaginal color Doppler study of endometrial blood flow changes. *Ultrasound Obstet. Gynecol.*, **2** (Suppl.), 82

3. Luzi, G., Margiacchi, P., Coata, G., Longo, A., Cucchia, G. C., Cosmi, E. V. and Direnzo, G. (1992). Doppler velocimetry of uterine arteries in spontaneous and artificially induced menopause. *Ultrasound Obstet. Gynecol.*, **2s**, 126

4. Lobo, R. A. and Speroff, L. (1994). International consensus conference on postmenopausal hormone therapy and the cardiovascular system. *Fertil. Steril.*, **61**(4), 592–5

5. Bonilla-Musoles, F., Ballester, M. J. and Carrera, J. M. (1992). La Menopausia. In *Doppler Color Transvaginal*. (Barcelona: Masson-Salvat, Publishers)

6. Bourne, T. H., Crayford, T., Reynolds, K., Hampson, J., Campbell, S. and Collins, W. P. (1992). Transvaginal color Doppler ultrasonography for the diagnosis of uterine cancer. *J. Ultrasound Med.*, **11s**, 33

7. Thaler, I., Manor, D., Brandes, G., Rottem, S. and Itskovtz, J. (1990). Basic principles and clinical application of the transvaginal Doppler duplex system in reproductive medicine. *J. In Vitro Fertil. Embryo Transfer*, **7**, 74–9

8. Bourne, T. H., Hillard, T. C., Whitehead, M. I., Crook, D. and Campbell, S. (1990). Oestrogens, arterial status, and postmenopausal women. *Lancet*, **335**, 1470–1

9. Gangar, K. F., Vyas, S., Whitehead, M. I. *et al.* (1991). Pulsatility index in internal carotid artery in relation to transdermal oestradiol. *Lancet*, **338**, 839

10. Hillard, T. C., Bourne, T. H., Whitehead, M. I. *et al.* (1992). Differential effects of transdermal estradiol and sequential progestogens on impedance to blood flow within the uterine arteries of postmenopausal women. *Fertil. Steril.*, **58**, 959–63

11. Pines, A., Fisman, E. and Ayalon, D. (1992). Long-term effects of hormone replacement therapy on Doppler-derived parameters of aortic flow in postmenopausal women. *Chest*, **102**, 1496–500

12. Bourne, T. H., Campbell, S., Whitehead, M. I. *et al.* (1990). Detection of endometrial cancer in postmenopausal women by transvaginal ultrasonography and color flow image. *Br. Med. J.*, **301**, 369

13. Bourne, T. H., Campbell, S., Steer, C. B., Royston, P., Whitehead, M. I. and Collins, W. P. (1991). Detection of endometrial cancer by transvaginal ultrasonography with color flow imaging and blood flow analysis: a preliminary report. *Gynecol. Oncol.*, **40**, 253–9

14. Zalud, I., Conway, C., Schulman, H. and Trinca, D. (1993). Endometrial and myometrial thickness and uterine blood flow in postmenopausal women. The influence of hormone replacement therapy. *J. Ultrasound Med.*, **12**, 737–42

15. Bonilla-Musoles, F., Marti, M. C., Ballester, M. J. *et al.* (1995). Normal uterine arterial blood flow in postmenopausal women assessed by transvaginal color Doppler ultrasonography. *J. Ultrasound Med.*, **14**, 491–4

16. Bonilla-Musoles, F., Marti, M. C., Ballester, M. J. *et al.* (1995). Normal uterine arterial blood flow in postmenopausal women assessed by transvaginal color Doppler sonography: the effect of hormone replacement therapy. *J. Ultrasound Med.*, **14**, 497–501

17. Bonilla-Musoles, F., Marti, M. C., Ballester, M. J. *et al.* (1995). Transvaginal color Doppler assessment of endometrial status in normal postmenopausal women: the effect of hormone replacement therapy. *J. Ultrasound Med.*, **14**, 503–7

18. Pirhonen, J. P., Vuento, M. H., Makinen, J. I. and Salmi, T. A. (1993). Long-term effects of hormone replacement therapy on the uterus and uterine circulation. *Am. J. Obstet. Gynecol.*, **168**, 620

19. Bourne, T. H., Hillard, T. C., Whitehead, M. I., Campbell, S. and Collins, W. P. (1991). Transvaginal ultrasonography with color flow imaging to monitor hormone replacement therapy in postmenopausal women. *Br. J. Radiol.*, **64**, 657–61

20. Stampfer, M. J. and Colditz, G. A. (1991). Oestrogen replacement therapy and coronary heart disease: a quantitative assessment of the epidemiological evidence. *Prev. Med.*, **20**, 47–63

21. Green, A. and Bain, C. (1991). Epidemiological overview of oestrogen replacement and cardiovascular disease. *Baillière's Clin. Endocrinol. Metab.*, **7**(1), 95–112

22. Bush, T. L., Barrett-Connor, E., Cowan, L. D., Criqui, M. H., Wallace, R. B., Suchindran, C. M., Troyler, H. A. and Rifkind, B. M. (1987). Cardiovascular mortality and noncontraceptive use of estrogen in women. Results from the Lipid

Research Clinics Programme Follow-up Study. *Circulation*, **75**, 1102–9

23. Penotti, M., Mencioni, T., Gabrieli, L., Farina, M., Castiglioni, E. and Polvani, F. (1993). Blood flow variations in internal carotid and middle cerebral arteries induced by postmenopausal hormone replacement therapy. *Am. J. Obstet. Gynecol.*, **169**, 1226–32

24. De Ziegler, D., Bessis, R. and Frydman, R. (1991). Vascular resistance of uterine arteries: physiological effects of estradiol and progesterone. *Fertil. Steril.*, **55**, 775–9

25. Haarbo, J., Hassager, C. and Jensen, S. B. (1991). Serum lipids, lipoproteins and apolipoproteins during postmenopausal estrogen replacement therapy combined with either 19-nortestosterone derivatives or 17-hydroxyprogesterone derivatives. *Am. J. Med.*, **90**, 584–9

26. Jensen, J., Nilas, L. and Christiansen, C. (1990). Influence of menopause on serum lipids and lipoproteins. *Maturitas*, **12**, 321–31

27. Nasri, M. N., Shepherd, J. H., Setchel, M. E., Lowe, D. G. and Chard, T. (1991). The role of vaginal scan in measurement of endometrial thickness in postmenopausal women. *Br. J. Obstet. Gynaecol.*, **98**, 470–5

28. Grandberg, S., Wilkland, M., Karlsson, B. *et al.* (1991). Endometrial thickness as measured by endovaginal ultrasound for identifying endometrial pathology. *Am. J. Obstet. Gynecol.*, **164**, 39

29. Kurjak, A., Shalan, A., Sosic, A., Benic, S., Zudenigo, D., Upesic, B. and Predanic, C. (1993). Endometrial carcinoma in postmenopausal women: evaluation by transvaginal color Doppler sonography. *Am. J. Obstet. Gynecol.*, **169**, 1597–1603

Sonohysterography of endometrial and related disorders

11

A. C. Fleischer, J. A. Cullinan and A. K. Parsons

INTRODUCTION

The recently developed technique of saline infusion within the endometrial lumen under sonographic guidance, termed sonohysterography, is becoming more frequently utilized, particularly in the gynecologist's office and/or sonographic suites. It provides a means to detect polypoid endometrial lesions, submucosal fibroids, adhesions and uterine malformations that affect the lumen.

Sonohysterography has an important role in evaluation of the patient with unexplained postmenopausal bleeding and in those patients in whom the endometrium is thickened or indistinct on transvaginal sonography (TVS). Polyps are enigmatic tumors apparently caused by resistance to progesterone-induced apoptosis or exposure to excess endogenous or exogenous estrogen. They typically are associated with intermenstrual bleeding, cramping, and/or infertility. Carcinomas may also be polypoid or arise within polyps[1]. Sonohysterography affords clear detection of the polyp and its pedicle. This is in contrast to a thickened endometrium as a result of endometrial hyperplasia and/or carcinoma.

Intraluminal fluid collections are frequently seen on TVS. Although they may be associated with endometrial cancer in some patients, they are more frequently associated with benign conditions such as cervical stenosis[2]. This 'natural sonohysterography' can be used to advantage to outline endometrial surfaces. This chapter will provide an overview to the clinical utility and limitations of sonohysterography and a discussion of the circumstances in which they should be ordered and used.

TECHNIQUE

With the more extensive use of TVS, the possibility of improved delineation of the endometrial lumen with intraluminal fluid instillation became possible[3–6]. The technique utilizes sterile saline as a negative (anechoic) contrast medium to outline the endometrial lumen under continuous TVS visualization[7].

Sonohysterography is primarily utilized for evaluation of endometrial polyps, assessing the presence and extent of submucosal fibroids, detection of uterine synechiae and in selected cases of uterine malformations that involve the endometrial lumen. The reader is referred to several excellent descriptions of the spectrum of sonographic findings with this technique[7,8].

Prior to saline instillation, the standard procedure for TVS is followed, including covering the probe with a condom and placement of the transvaginal probe within the vaginal fornix and mid-vagina in order to delineate optimally the endometrial interfaces in both long and short axes. The images should be recorded on hard copy film or paper and videotape for later review.

Sonohysterography involves placement of a catheter into the uterine lumen through the endocervical canal. Catheter choices which can be utilized include insemination catheter, pediatric Foley, pediatric feeding tube or a plastic hysterosalpingogram (HSG) catheter (Figure 1). The pediatric feeding catheter is preferred, since it can be introduced easily into the cervix without much pain or discomfort. The balloon catheter is recommended when trying to evaluate tubal patency after assessment of uterine

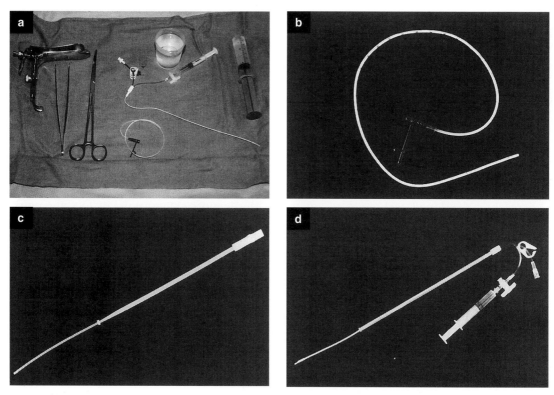

Figure 1 Set-up for sonohysterography: (a) set-up used for sonohysterography consisting of long straight forceps, open-lipped speculum, pediatric feeding catheter, HSG catheter with inflatable balloon tip, saline, long Q-tip, and cleansing solution. Catheters used for sonohysterography: (b) pediatric feeding tube with centimeter markers; (c) insemination catheter. This is stiffer than the pediatric feeding catheters; a plastic collar around the catheter indicates depth of placement, usually placed at 7 cm from the tip; (d) H/S HSG catheter with inflatable balloon

lumen patency. Once the cervix is cleansed with a cleansing solution and stabilized with a speculum, 3–10 cm^3 of sterile saline is injected under sonographic visualization. The slow instillation of saline, allowing reflux out of the cervix, also diminishes the possibility of pain during instillation. The endometrium is imaged in both long and short axis, with specific attention to its regularity and thickness (Figure 2).

The procedure is best performed in the early follicular phase. This avoids confusing images arising from mildly irregular secretory endometrium or clots that may be encountered in the late secretory portion of the cycle and also decreases the possibility of dislodging an unsuspected early pregnancy. Since endometrial polyps are echogenic, the relatively hypoechoic proliferative phase endometrium is best shown against the relatively hyperechoic proliferative phase endometrium (Figures 3 and 4). Conversely, submucosal fibroids may best be imaged in the secretory phase since they are typically hypoechoic and their relation to the displaced endometrium may be best delineated during this phase of the cycle (Figure 5).

Contraindications to sonohysterography include hematometra, extensive pelvic inflammatory disease, or significant cervical stenosis. Rarely an atrophic or stenotic vagina from aging or previous radiation therapy can produce significant discomfort even with placement of the vaginal speculum.

Typically, the patient does not experience significant discomfort if the catheter is properly placed in the fundus and only small amounts of fluid are gently infused and allowed to reflux out of the cervix. Prophylactic antibiotics are usually not needed but preprocedural non-steroidal

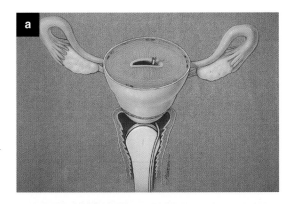

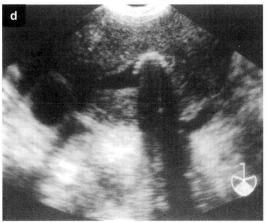

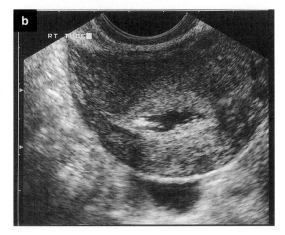

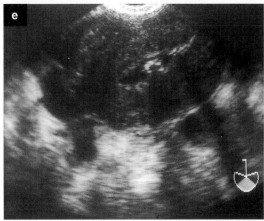

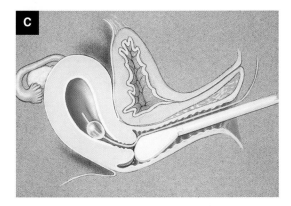

Figure 2 Normal sonohysterography: (a) diagram showing pediatric feeding tube used for sonohysterography. The tip should be advanced into the fundus to obtain maximal dilatation. (b) Transvaginal sonogram during initial fluid instillation showing secretory phase endometrium. The catheter produces a linear artifact within the lumen. (c) Diagram of sonohysterography using pediatric Foley with inflatable balloon. The inflated balloon obstructs reflux, allowing better luminal distension in some patients with relatively patalous cervix. (d, e) TVS showing same balloon when inflated (d) and deflated (e)

anti-inflammatories are helpful to minimize uterine cramping.

TYPICAL SONOGRAPHIC FINDINGS

The intraluminal surface of the normal endometrium is usually delineated in its entirety after the introduction of intraluminal fluid. On short axis, the normal areas of endometrial invagination in both tubal ostia can be seen. In general, the endometrium measures up to 4 mm in thickness per single layer and should have a relatively regular and homogeneous texture. The secretory phase endometrium is mildly irregular and may contain 'endometrial wrinkles' a few

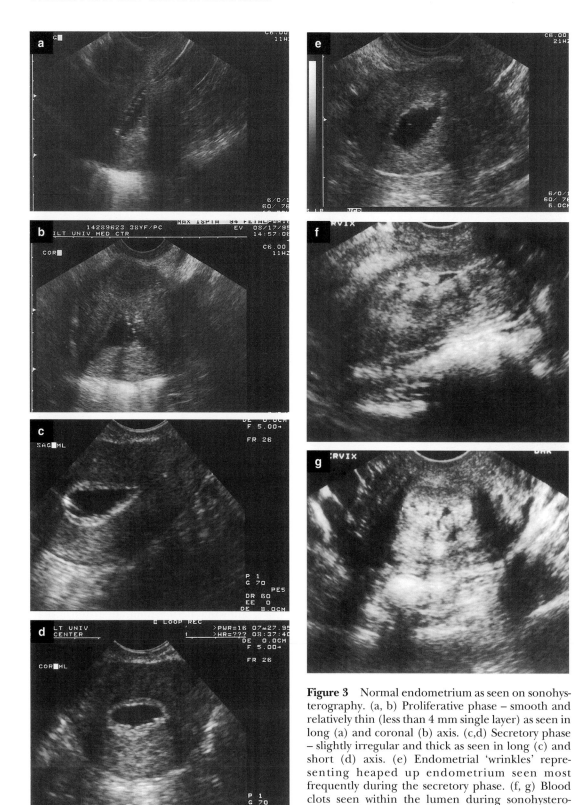

Figure 3 Normal endometrium as seen on sonohysterography. (a, b) Proliferative phase – smooth and relatively thin (less than 4 mm single layer) as seen in long (a) and coronal (b) axis. (c,d) Secretory phase – slightly irregular and thick as seen in long (c) and short (d) axis. (e) Endometrial 'wrinkles' representing heaped up endometrium seen most frequently during the secretory phase. (f, g) Blood clots seen within the lumen during sonohysterography on long (f) and short (g) axis

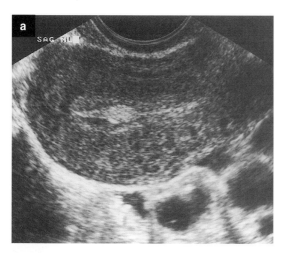 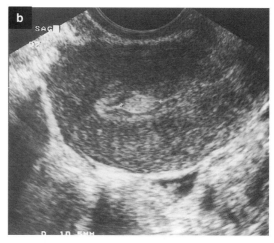

Figure 4 Sonographically apparent polyp. (a) Sagittal TVS showing polyp separating endometrial surfaces. (b) Same patient as in (a); the cleavage produced by the polyp (between cursors) separating the two endometrial layers is seen

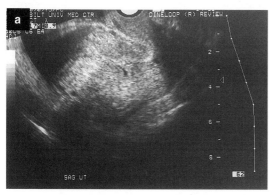 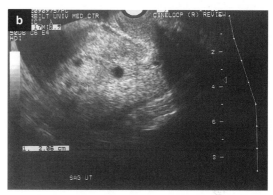

Figure 5 Sonographically nearly inapparent polyp. (a) TVS showing a large polyp occupying a markedly enlarged endometrial lumen. Only a sliver of fluid is seen surrounding this polyp which on histology contained a focus of clear-cell carcinoma. (b) Short-axis view showing near conspicuity of polyp with surrounding myometrium

millimeters in height. The endometrium is typically similar in thickness and texture, but focal irregularities can be observed in some patients.

Polyps

Endometrial polyps are typically echogenic and project into the endometrial lumen (Figures 5 and 6). Larger polyps may contain cystic spaces representing obstructed glands within the polyp. In the non-distended endometrium, they typically displace the median echo which may represent refluxed cervical mucus and are best seen just before ovulation (Figure 4). As they

enlarge, they can distend the cavity and may be apparent without iatrogenic distension of the endometrial lumen. Some are outlined by trapped intraluminal fluid, mucus, or blood. The vascularity of the pedicle can be demonstrated in some cases (Figure 7).

Submucosal fibroids

Submucosal fibroids are typically hypoechoic and displace the basalis layer of the endometrium (Figure 8). The amount of extension into the myometrial layers is important to determine;

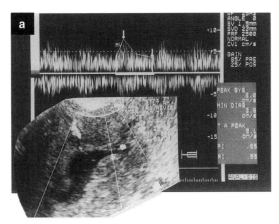

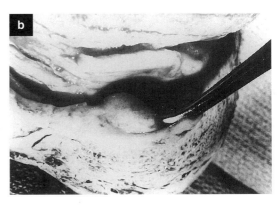

Figure 6 Polyp with color Doppler sonography showing vascularity. (a) Combined transvaginal sonogram and Doppler spectrum from vessel within polyp showing low impedance flow and (b) sectioned uterus showing polyp

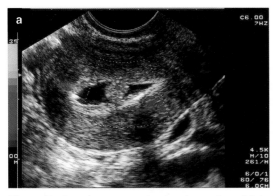

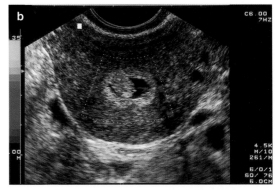

Figure 7 Sonohysterography showing polyp with its vascularity shown on color Doppler sonography. (a) In the sagittal plane, the power Doppler shows vascularity within the pedicle of the polyp. (b) The same as in (a) in the coronal plane

superficial submucosal fibroids with a thin stalk may be removed by wire loop or alligator forceps whereas those that extend beyond the endometrial–myometrial interface will not be amenable to wire loop resection.

Synechiae

Synechiae typically occur as the sequelae of intrauterine instrumentation. They may be either echogenic or hypoechoic depending on their fibrous content (Figure 9). The hypoechoic synechiae are best delineated in the background of the typically echogenic secretory phase endometrium[9].

Other findings

Certain uterine malformations that affect the lumen such as bicornuate or septate uteri may be evaluated using sonohysterography. The presence or absence of a fundal cleft is important in distinguishing bicornuate uteri from septated uteri (Figure 10).

Color Doppler sonography may be helpful to identify the vascular pedicle of a polyp as well as the vascular rim of certain leiomyomata (Figure 7). Sonohysterography is helpful in determining whether a polyp has a wide or narrow pedicle since those with a thin pedicle are more easily removed with a forceps in the office than ones with a thick pedicle.

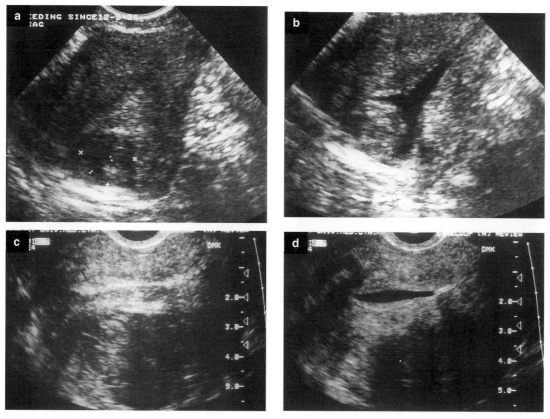

Figure 8 Submucosal fibroid: (a) prior to sonohysterography, the hypoechoic submucosal fibroid is seen to displace overlying echogenic endometrium; (b) after saline instillation, the overlying endometrium and submucosal leiomyoma are seen. Intramural fibroid: (c) prior to sonohysterography, an intramural leiomyoma is seen extending into the outer layer of myometrium; (d) after saline instillation, the relationship of the normal endometrium to the intramural leiomyoma is clearly demonstrated

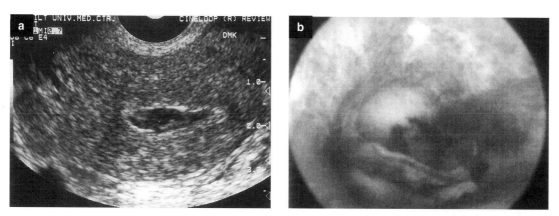

Figure 9 Adhesions: (a) sonohysterography showing linear adhesions crossing lumen; (b) hysteroscopy shows the adhesion (courtesy of Dr E. Eisenberg)

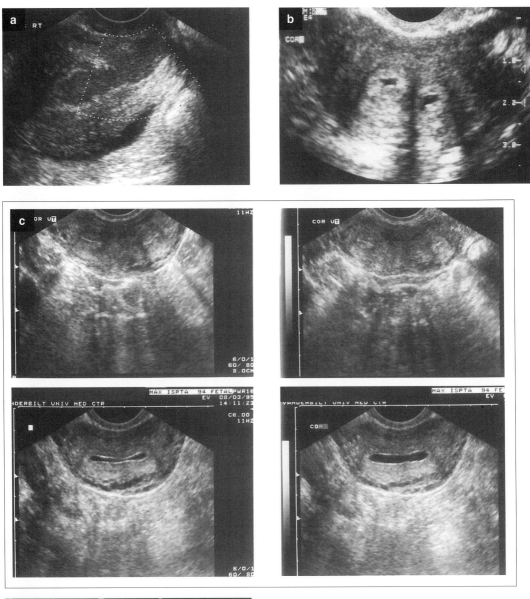

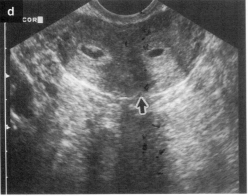

Figure 10 Miscellaneous conditions: (a) hematometra, pre-sonohysterography TVS showed hematometra, a contraindication to sonohysterography; (b) septate uterus: sonohysterography showed two lumina separated by a thick septum. There was no fundal cleft; (c, d) bicornuate uterus: sonohysterography showing two endometrial lumina but, in contrast to (b), a fundal cleft (arrowhead) is seen. Composite TVS pre- and post-saline instillation. Two endometrial lumina are seen prior to (top) and after (bottom) saline instillation. (d) The two endometrial lumina are seen best on this coronal TVS taken through the fundus. The fundal cleft (arrow) is seen on this image

Sonohysterography is also particularly·helpful in determining whether certain intraluminal cystic areas are within a polyp or the myometrium. Punctate cystic spaces are frequently seen within polyps as a result of glandular obstruc-tion. They may also be seen within the myometrium in women who are on tamoxifen, possibly as a result of reactivation of dormant adenomyosis[5]

References

1. Salm, R. (1972). The incidence and significance of early carcinomas in endometrial polyps. *J. Pathol.*, **108**, 47–53
2. Pardo, J., Kaplan, B., Nitke, S., Ovadia, J., Segal, J. and Neri, A. (1994). Postmenopausal intrauterine fluid collection: correlation between ultrasound and hysteroscopy. *Ultrasound Obstet. Gynecol.*, **4**, 224–6
3. Syrop, C. H. and Sahakian, V. (1992). Transvaginal sonographic detection of endometrial polyps with fluid contrast augmentation. *Obstet. Gynecol.*, **79**, 1041–3
4. Parsons, A. K. and Lense, J. J. (1993). Sonohysterography for endometrial abnormalities: preliminary results. *J. Clin. Ultrasound*, **21**, 87–95
5. Goldstein, S. R. (1994). Unusual ultrasonographic appearance of the uterus in patients receiving tamoxifen. *Am. J. Obstet. Gynecol.*, **170**, 447–51
6. Dubinsky, T., Parvey, H., Gormaz, G. and Maklad, N. (1995). Transvaginal hysterosonography in the evaluation of small endometrial masses. *J. Ultrasound Med.*, **14**, 1–6
7. Cullinan, J., Fleischer, A., Kepple, D. and Arnold, A. (1995). Sonohysterography: a technique for endometrial evaluation. *Radiographics*, **15**, 501–14
8. Parsons, A., Cullinan, J. A., Goldstein, S. and Fleischer, A. C. (1995). Sonohysterography, sonosalpingography and sonohysterosalpingography. In Fleischer, A., Romero, R. and Manning, R. (eds.) *Sonography in Obstetrics and Gynecology*, pp. 931–68. (Stamford, CT: Appleton Lange)
9. Narayan, R. and Goswamy, R. K. (1993). Transvaginal sonography of the uterine cavity with hysteroscopic correlation in the investigation of infertility. *Ultrasound Obstet. Gynecol.*, **3**, 129–33

Transabdominal and transvaginal pulsed and color Doppler sonography of adenomyosis

12

M. Hirai

INTRODUCTION

The diagnosis of adenomyosis of the uterus has been made by the classic clinical symptoms of dysmenorrhea and/or hypermenorrhea with enlarged uterus. Recent reports suggest that hormonal therapies are often effective in the treatment of adenomyosis, and, therefore, sonographic identification of adenomyosis and its differential diagnosis are necessary.

Although there are several reported etiologies, pathologically, adenomyosis is defined as the abnormal distribution of nests of histologically benign endometrial tissue in the myometrium and it may be focal or diffuse[1]. In adenomyosis, the uterine enlargement is usually moderate; therefore transvaginal sonography (TVS) with a high-frequency transducer, 5.0 MHz or higher, is superior to transabdominal sonography (TAS) in order to obtain a better resolution of the uterine structure. However, TAS may be necessary when the uterus is extremely enlarged, for example, due to coexisting myoma.

IDENTIFICATION OF ADENOMYOSIS

The typical features of adenomyosis are:

(1) Thickened myometrium;

(2) Asymmetrical uterus;

(3) Abnormal myometrial texture;

(4) Absent or irregular contour;

(5) Abnormal endometrium.

Thickened myometrium and asymmetrical uterus

Because of ectopic growth of endometrium in the uterus, thickening of the myometrium is often observed in adenomyosis. Bohman and co-workers report thickening of the posterior of the uterus in five of seven cases of adenomyosis[2]. The increase in size produced by adenomyosis is of diffuse type, and usually one wall, the posterior, is much thicker than the other[3]. In our experience, adenomyosis involves either the posterior wall (63%) of the uterus or the anterior wall (27%) predominantly and only occasionally are both walls involved (10%). Consequently, the uterus is often asymmetrical (Figures 1 and 2).

To evaluate the enlargement and asymmetry of the uterus, the following measurements are

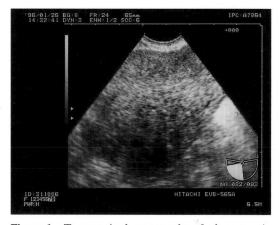

Figure 1 Transvaginal sonography of adenomyosis: a honeycomb pattern is seen in the center of the posterior wall of the uterus

useful: the maximal myometrial thickness in the uterine fundus (Mf); and the maximal myometrial thickness in the uterine body (Mb) (only the myometrium was measured. Fleischer and co-workers previously suggested endometrial changes in spontaneous cycles[4]); also, the ratio (R) of Mb to the opposite side myometrial thickness (Mo). If myoma exists (the differential diagnosis will be discussed later), the measurement is made excluding it. Figure 3 shows the method of the measurements. Our data (Table 1) suggest that Mf > 22 mm, Mb > 28 mm, and/or R > 1.4 should be considered a sign of adenomyosis[5].

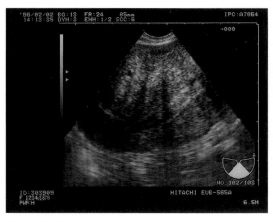

Figure 2 Transvaginal sonography of adenomyosis: several irregular cysts are seen

Abnormal myometrial texture

Walsh and co-workers report that the focal honeycomb pattern and/or 5–7 mm irregular cystic spaces are often identified in the normal echo pattern of the uterus[6]. A focal honeycomb pattern in hyperechoic lesion is seen in Figure 1. Several irregular cystic spaces in hyperechoic lesions are seen in Figure 2. The cystic spaces are often less than 5 mm or very small. It is difficult to identify those very small cysts sonographically. It is necessary to change the scan angles to see the cystic spaces from different directions. Artifacts or vessels should be differentiated from them. Color flow imaging and/or pulsed Doppler may also be helpful to differentiate vessels from the cystic spaces (Figure 4).

The myometrial texture is often hyperechoic; however, it may be normal, hypoechoic or mixed.

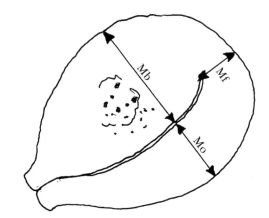

Figure 3 Measurements of the uterine myometrium: Mf, maximal myometrial thickness in the uterine fundus; Mb, maximal myometrial thickness in the uterine body; Mo, the thickness of the myometrium of the opposite side of Mb; R, Mb/Mo

Table 1 Measurements of myometrial thickness and ratio; mean ± SD (range)

	n	Mf (mm)	Mb (mm)	R
Adenomyosis	32	27.0 ± 16.0 (18–83)	41.6 ± 14.5 (19–85)	2.3 ± 1.6 (1.0–9.4)
Adenomyosis with myoma	30	26.2 ± 11.0 (5–49)	33.7 ± 11.4 (10–55)	1.7 ± 0.5 (1.0–2.9)
Myoma	26	12.1 ± 3.9 (6–22)	17.5 ± 3.9 (9–27)	1.1 ± 0.1 (1.0–1.4)
CIS (cervical cancer) or uterine prolapse as control	20	13.1 ± 3.2 (9–18)	19.3 ± 3.8 (13–25)	1.0 ± 0.03 (1.0–1.1)

Mf, maximal myometrial thickness in the uterine fundus; Mb, maximal myometrial thickness in the uterine body; R, Mb/Mo (myometrial thickness of the opposite side of the wall); CIS, carcinoma *in situ*

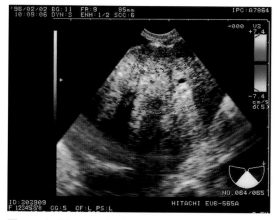

Figure 4 Transvaginal color flow image of adenomyosis: no flow is demonstrated in the cyst

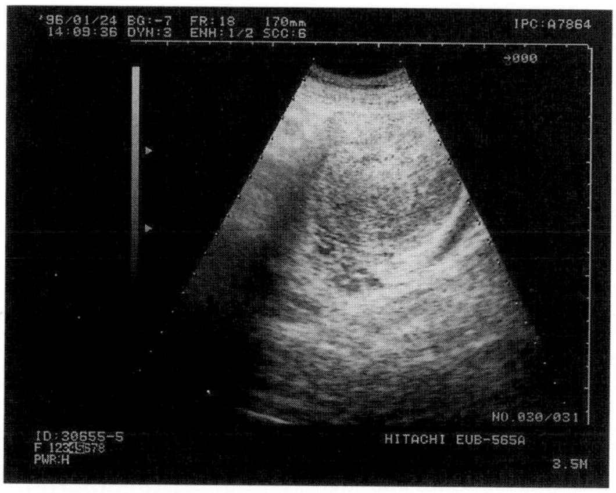

Figure 5 Transvaginal sonography of myoma: a round, smooth contour of the myoma is seen

Absent or irregular contour

In the diffuse type of adenomyosis, contour is often absent (Figure 2), while irregular contour may be seen both in the diffuse type (Figure 1) and the focal type. On the other hand, a round smooth contour is usually seen around myoma (Figure 5). This is an important aspect of the differential diagnosis between adenomyosis and myoma. With color flow imaging, it is often possible to see feeding vessels surrounding myoma or sarcoma.

To obtain the whole image of feeding vessels, transabdominal sonography is superior to transvaginal sonography. Figure 6 shows the surrounding vessels of the tumor. However, no surrounding vessels are seen in Figures 4 and 7 (adenomyosis).

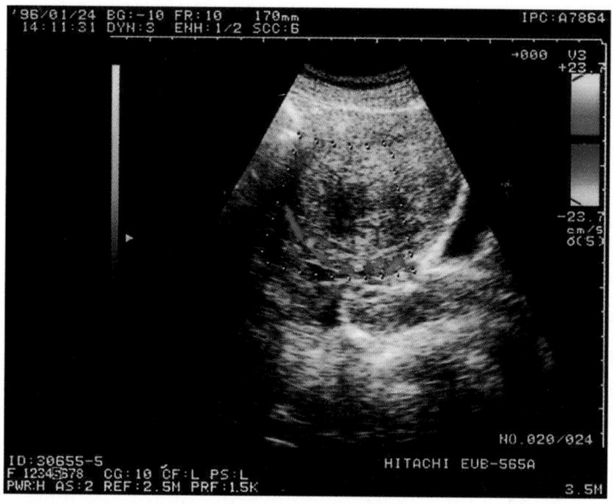

Abnormal endometrium

Irregular and/or compressed endometrium is seen in adenomyosis. The endometrial irregularity is usually subtle; sometimes endometrial defects (diverticula-like changes) are visualized (Figures 7 and 8) or the endometrial layer may look normal. Other diseases which cause irregular endometrium include endometrial cancer, endometrial hyperplasia, endometritis, endometrial polyps and hematometria. Endometrial hyperplasia is sometimes associated with adenomyosis. Myoma and sarcoma as well as adenomyosis compress the endometrium.

Figure 6 Transabdominal color flow image of myoma: a feeding artery is circulating around the myoma

Several conditions may be responsible for the endometrial abnormality; therefore differential diagnosis is important.

DIFFERENTIAL DIAGNOSIS

Adenomyosis and myoma

The differentiation of adenomyosis from myoma is discussed above.

Adenomyosis and uterine malignancies

Differentiating adenomyosis from uterine malignancies or detecting coexisting uterine

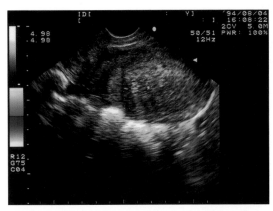

Figure 7 Transvaginal sonography of adenomyosis: several signals from somewhat hyperechoic myometrium are seen. Irregular endometrium is also visualized

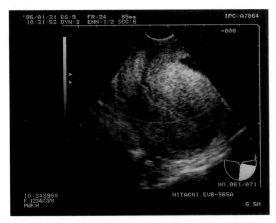

Figure 8 Transvaginal sonography of adenomyosis: irregular endometrium is visualized. Endometrial defects (diverticula-like changes) are seen

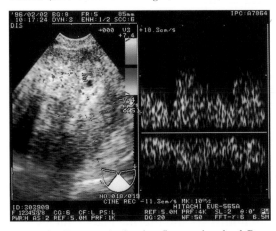

Figure 9 Transvaginal color flow and pulsed Doppler image of adenomyosis. The spectral analysis indicates a benign condition (RI = 0.61, V_{max} = 10.2 cm/s)

Table 2 RI and V_{max} for adenomyosis, myoma and uterine malignancies: mean ± SD (range)

	n	RI	V_{max} (cm/s)
Adenomyosis	35	0.57 ± 0.08 (0.43–0.78)	14.1 ± 4.1 (7.6–25.3)
Myoma (< 6 cm)	27	0.56 ± 0.07 (0.39–0.68)	17.0 ± 4.8 (9.6–28.7)
Uterine malignancies	9	0.40 ± 0.05 (0.33–0.51)	29.8 ± 7.8 (19.6–41.1)

RI, resistance index; V_{max}, peak systolic velocity

malignancy is very important especially when patients are candidates for hormonal therapy. Basically, the endometrial change is rather irregular and diverticulum-like in adenomyosis, while the change is proliferative in endometrial cancer. However, it should be noted that adenomyosis is encountered more frequently in uteri with endometrial cancer than in those without and adenomyosis is usually more extensive in the presence of endometrial cancer[7]. In our findings, adenomyosis was associated with endometrial hyperplasia in 23% (31/134), with atypical endometrial hyperplasia in 13% (17/134), and with endometrial cancer in 3% (4/134). Therefore, gray-scale TVS findings may sometimes be ambiguous. Color and pulsed Doppler analyses are often useful to differentiate adenomyosis (Figure 9) from uterine malignancies. Our color Doppler study suggests a significant difference between adenomyosis and uterine malignancies (endometrial cancer, sarcoma, cervical cancer)[8].

Table 2 shows the results of 71 patients (age range 37–83 years old) examined using a 6.5-MHz transvaginal probe. Patients who were pregnant or under hormonal therapy were not included. Premenopausal patients were scanned during the proliferative days of a cycle (days 6 to 10). At least three intratumoral vessels were examined and the lowest resistance index (RI) and the V_{max} (highest peak systolic velocity) were recorded. There were statistically significant differences between adenomyosis and uterine malignancies both in RI and V_{max} ($p < 0.001$, $p < 0.001$, Mann–Whitney U test). Although there were some false-negative cases, our results suggest that a low RI (< 0.43) and/or a high V_{max} (> 23.5 cm/s) should be considered a sign of malignancy. Inflammatory and/or degenerative conditions of the uterus may affect the results. Also, some drugs (e.g. vasodilators) affect the uterine hemodynamics. Possible preparations should be made before scans. For the management of borderline cases, frequent follow-up scans with or without the hormonal therapy, biopsy, or operation may be necessary.

ACKNOWLEDGEMENTS

I would like to thank Hitach Medical Corporation and Aloka Co. Ltd for their assistance in this research.

References

1. Kraus, F. T. (1990). Female genitalia. In Kissane, J. M. (ed.) *Anderson's Pathology*, pp. 1663–4. (St. Louis: Mosby)
2. Bohman, M. E., Ensor, R. E. and Sanders, R. C. (1987). Sonographic findings in adenomyosis of the uterus. *Am. J. Roentgenol.*, **148**, 765–6
3. Novak, E. R. and Woodruff, J. D. (1979). Adenomyosis. In Novak, E. R. and Woodruff, J. D. (eds.) *Novak's Gynecologic and Obstetric Pathology with Clinical and Endocrine Relations*, 8th edn., pp. 261–71. (Philadelphia: Sanders)
4. Fleischer, A. C., Kalemeris, G. C. and Entman, S. S. (1986). Sonographic depiction of the endometrium during normal cycles. *Ultrasound Med. Biol.*, **12**, 271–7
5. Hirai, M., Ookubo, H., Inaba, N. and Takamizawa, H. (1993). A study for the diagnosis of adenomyosis by TVS. *Chiba Med. J.*, **69**, 25–45
6. Walsh, J. W., Taylor, K. J. W. and Rosenfield, A. T. (1979). Gray scale ultrasonography in the diagnosis of endometriosis and adenomyosis. *Am. J. Roentgenol.*, **132**, 87–90
7. Marcus, C. C. (1961). Relationships of adenomyosis uteri to endometrial hyperplasia and endometrial carcinoma. *Am. J. Obstet. Gynecol.*, **82**, 408–16
8. Hirai, M., Shibata, K., Sagai, H., Sekiya, S. and Goldberg, B. B. (1995). Transvaginal pulsed and color Doppler sonography for the evaluation of adenomyosis. *J. Ultrasound Med.*, **14**, 529–32

Guidance with transrectal sonography for operative procedures involving endometrial disorders 13

A. C. Fleischer

Transrectal sonography can provide guidance for endometrial biopsy and/or dilatation and curettage. It can also be used during hysteroscopy as a means to guide biopsy or polyp removal[1]. The bi-plane transrectal probe is recommended since one can image in the sagittal plane as well as axially, thereby confirming the position of a biopsy catheter or curette in two planes (Figures 1 and 2). Transrectal sonography is particularly helpful in patients whose external cervical os cannot be adequately visualized due to vaginal stenosis or extensive cervical cancer, for example.

The biplane transrectal probe is covered with a condom and fluid is introduced within the condom. The covered probe is introduced into the rectum after KY jelly is spread over the tip and anterior surface of the condom. This provides optimal contact with the rectal wall. The cervix is usually imaged initially in the longitudinal plane followed by selected images in the axial orientation.

If one is interested in localization of the external os, the endocervical canal can be identified on longitudinal views (Figure 3). Once the dilator is introduced into the cervix,

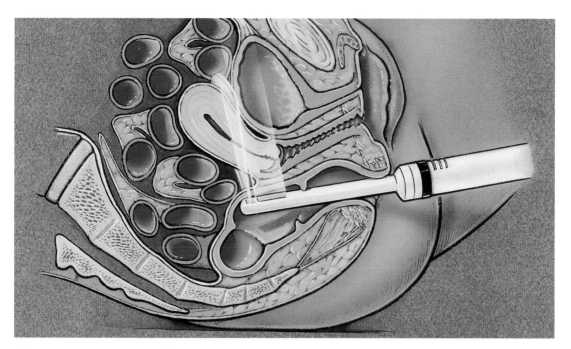

Figure 1 Diagram showing transrectal sonography of the cervix and endometrium in the long axis; the cervix and upper vagina are depicted

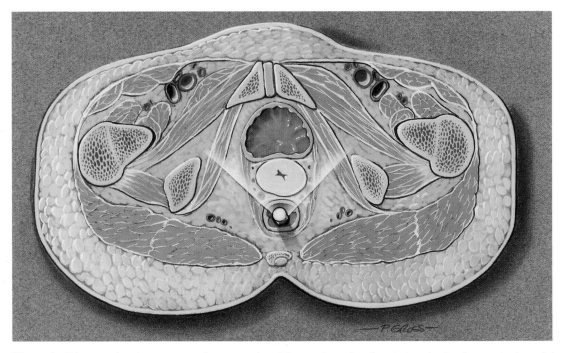

Figure 2 Diagram showing transrectal sonography of the cervix and endometrium in the short axis: the axial plane of the lower uterus and cervix can be depicted

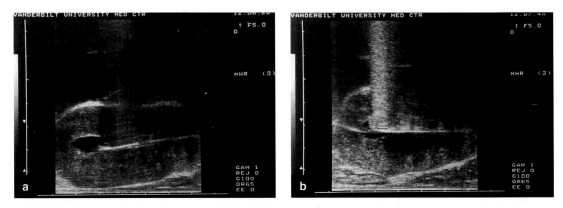

Figure 3 Transrectal sonographic guidance of D & C: (a) initially, the posterior layer of endometrium is curettaged; (b) after redirection of the curettage anteriorly, the anterior layer of endometrium is sampled

its central location can be confirmed with the axial scan. If perforation is suspected, it can be documented with transrectal sonography (Figure 4).

We have had experience with over 25 cases where transrectal sonography was useful in guiding dilatation and curettage, intrauterine tandem placement, or cerclage suture place-

ment[2]. Transrectal sonography can also be used for guiding biopsy or aspiration of suspicious areas of endometrial irregularity or thickening[3,4].

If it is used intraoperatively, the transducer is held by the operator and a sterile towel is placed over the operator's hand. The retractors are placed to the side walls of the vagina

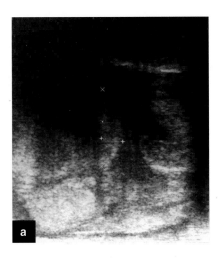
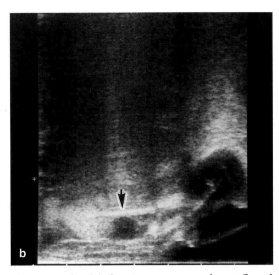

Figure 4 Uterine perforation documented by transrectal sonography: (a) the uterus was severely anteflexed (the cursors outline the endometrium); (b) upon introduction of the dilator it extended into a bowel loop within the cul-de-sac (arrowhead)

allowing ultrasound to be transmitted through the rectum in a long-axis plane. The study should be videotaped for documentation purposes.

We have observed a few cases of uterine perforation. The dilator and/or tandem could be identified as being extrauterine in both cases.

References

1. Shalev, E. (1994). Ultrasound controlled operative hysteroscopy. *J. Am. Coll. Surg.*, **179**, 70
2. Fleischer, A., Burnett, L., Jones, H. and Cullinan, J. (1995). Transrectal and transperineal sonography for guided intrauterine procedures. *J. Ultrasound Med.*, **14**, 135–8
3. Savader, B., Hamper, U., Sheth, S., Ballard, R. and Sarden, R. (1990). Pelvic masses: aspiration biopsy with transrectal sonography. *Radiology*, **176**, 351–3
4. Alexander, A., Eschelman, D. and Nazarian, L. (1994). Transrectal sonographically guided drainage of deep pelvic abscesses. *Am. J. Roentgenol.*, **112**, 1227

Transvaginal sonography of the endometrium and predictors of clinical outcome after transcervical resection of the endometrium

14

O. Istre

INTRODUCTION

Menstrual disturbances are common in fertile and premenopausal women and menorrhagia is the most common cause of iron deficiency in these patients[1,2]. Some of these problems are transient[3,4] and many patients are treated effectively in general practice[5,6]. When medical therapy fails, hysterectomy has been the only surgical alternative[7] and represents the most commonly performed major operation for women of reproductive age[8,9]. This operation implies a hospital stay of about 1 week, and subsequent sick leave of 4–6 weeks. The overall mortality rate is 16.1 per 10 000 operations[10] and the complication rate (including minor complications) 43% and 25% after abdominal and vaginal hysterectomy, respectively[11]. However, today even hysterectomy has been modified with endoscopic methods for removal of the uterus. These methods imply shorter hospital stays and faster convalescence[12]. Still, however, there is research into alternative, less invasive procedures such as transcervical techniques for isolated removal of the endometrium to decrease menstrual bleeding. Transcervical resection of the endometrium (TCRE) has become widely used for the treatment of menorrhagia[13,14], and a detailed knowledge of the postoperative appearance of the uterus is important for the correct management of these patients. Second-look hysteroscopy has shown that the cavity is transformed into a narrow fibrotic tube after the operation[14,15]. Other methods currently used for the characterization of uterine morphology include transvaginal ultrasound examination (transvaginal sonography; TVS). TVS has previously been used to show a decrease in uterine dimensions after TCRE in about 50% of patients studied[16]. However, of particular relevance to the procedure of TCRE is whether the day of the menstrual cycle on which it is done, the presence of fibroids, or thick endometrium alter the clinical outcome. TVS could then be used to select more accurately those women who would benefit from the procedure, and perhaps time surgery more effectively regarding the patient's menses or drug therapy to achieve endometrial thinning. TVS was performed in patients undergoing TCRE with particular attention being given to the presence or absence of fibroids, the preoperative endometrial thickness, and the presence or absence of residual endometrium or cavity fluid after surgery.

Preoperative investigation

Prior to TCRE, 188 patients underwent TVS by using General Electric® RT 2800 (GE, London, UK), or Aloka® 3500 ultrasound unit (Aloka Co Ltd, Tokyo, Japan) equipped with a 5-MHz vaginal probe.

The purpose of TVS was to test the possible predictive value for a clinical outcome of endometrial thickness (both layers, from one endo-myometrial interface to the other) and anteroposterior diameters (measured as the largest diameter oblique to the endometrium)

(Figure 1). An endometrial thickness of 8.0 mm was picked as a cut-off limit because this divided the groups into comparative study populations and represented the mean value. The presence or absence of submucous fibroids were noted and their number and largest diameters recorded. The operation was scheduled despite the menstrual cycle. An endometrial biopsy (Pipelle courniere, Prodimed®, France)[17,18] and a cervical smear by means of Kollstad's spatula (A. Knutsen®, Norway) and cytobrush (Rocket of London®, UK) were taken.

Postoperative follow-up

TVS was performed and the anteroposterior diameter of the uterus was assessed on each postoperative visit. Furthermore, the thickness of residual endometrium, if any, was measured. Residual endometrium on TVS was defined as areas of different gray scale in the fundus and the largest diameter was measured. Collections of fluid indicative of hematometra were looked for and their dimensions noted. The patients were seen 6 weeks after surgery to evaluate the immediate effects of the procedure, in particular fever, pain and vaginal discharge. The women were seen again at 6 months to identify treatment failures so that further treatment could be planned. Follow-up bleeding pattern and menstrual pain were assessed using the same scores as preoperatively.

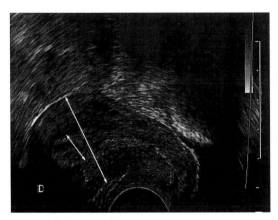

Figure 1 Anteroposterior diameter (long arrow) and endometrial thickness (short arrow) of the uterus

UTERINE MORPHOLOGY AFTER TCRE

Variable amounts of endometrium were found in 87% of the patients undergoing second-look hysteroscopy after 1 year by histological examination of random biopsies[14]. The amount of residual endometrium was consistently underestimated at the hysteroscopic examination. At TVS, the number of patients with detectable endometrium eventually increased from 15% after 6 weeks to 38% after a year. Taken together, the data available suggest that small nests of endometrium are left behind in the vast majority of patients after TCRE, in some patients probably because of adenomyosis. Some proliferation seems to occur during the 1st year after TCRE, despite the continued experience of a satisfactory clinical result.

Patients with histologically verified endometrium covering more than 50% of the surface area experienced more bleeding than patients with less than 50% after 1 year. This is in contrast to the finding in women with intact endometrium showing no correlation between the endometrial surface area and the menstrual volume[19]. However, both groups had marked reduction in bleeding after the operation, and residual endometrium was also found in some patients with amenorrhea after TCRE.

Retention of fluid and cervical stenosis

Transvaginal sonography 1 year after TCRE in 188 out of 195 consecutive patients revealed retention of fluid in 13 (7%)[20]. Two of these (15%) experienced severe dysmenorrhea, indicating significant cervical stenosis. Retention of fluid may thus occur without clinical signs of cervical stenosis, but pain after TCRE motivates TVS to exclude hematometra.

PREDICTORS OF CLINICAL OUTCOME

Multivariate analysis was applied to the total clinical series ($n = 412$) to define the possible predictive value of operators' experience, occurrence of fibroids, metrorrhagia, previous sterilization, patients' age, dysmenorrhea and suspicion of adenomyosis at histological examination of the resected tissue. Moreover, the predictive value of endometrial thickness and uterine anteroposterior diameter was evaluated in 188 patients[21].

Operators' experience

Operators' experience was the most important predictor of a positive result as for patients' satisfaction, amenorrhea, reduced postoperative pain and risk of reresection and hysterectomy[21], in parallel to the significance of this parameter for the complication rate.

Metrorrhagia

Some studies have restricted the use of endometrial resection to patients with pure menorrhagia[14]. Patients with metrorrhagia were included in the present study and seemed to experience a higher amenorrhea rate (65% versus 44%, $p = 0.051$) compared with patients with menorrhagia, while only three of 41 patients had irregular bleeding in the control group. Thus, no evidence was found that these patients have a less satisfactory effect with TCRE.

Dysmenorrhea and adenomyosis

Identical dysmenorrhea frequency was found prior to operation (59%) independent of preoperative endometrial thickness or histological phase found at operation. However, significant pain reduction was obtained on 12 months' follow-up; only 19 (10%) women complained of dysmenorrhea or pain. It is a general belief that adenomyosis may cause menorrhagia and dysmenorrhea, but firm evidence has been difficult to obtain. Early postmortem studies revealed an overall incidence of 54%, showing that many cases are asymptomatic[22]. Analysis of 212 patients undergoing hysterectomy failed to reveal any symptoms specific to adenomyosis[23]. However, a direct relation between myometrial invasion and severity of dysmenorrhea had also been reported[24]. Some evidence suggests that

women with dysmenorrhea and menorrhagia were less satisfied after TCRE than those with menorrhagia alone[25]. Patients with adenomyosis more often complained of dysmenorrhea. Moreover, adenomyosis seemed to represent a predictor of subsequent risk of hysterectomy after TCRE, although these patients often showed a mixed pathology with adenomyosis and fibroids[21]. Still, however, a satisfactory overall clinical improvement was observed. Removal of the endometrium through TCRE would be expected to decrease the output of prostaglandin, thus decreasing myometrial hypercontractility and dysmenorrheic pain. Also superficial adenomyosis (grade I adenomyosis[26]), which extends to the superficial parts of the myometrium, should be removed by TCRE. In accordance, TCRE produced pain relief in most patients whether or not adenomyosis was diagnosed in the resected tissue.

Age

Young age was associated with a less satisfactory result, a lower incidence of amenorrhea and more postoperative pain. Amenorrhea induced by the menopause should by itself improve overall clinical results at follow-up of the older patient[14,25]. So far, it would seem that endometrial resection should largely be avoided in young women.

Previous sterilization

Previous sterilization was, however, also a predictor of pain after TCRE. It is possible that some of these patients experience the post-ablation-tubal sterilization syndrome, caused by medial tubal accumulation of blood originating from residual cornual endometrium, as described after roller-ball coagulation[27]. TVS would be of great value in the diagnosis of these patients.

Fibroids

Patients with fibroids had a lower incidence of amenorrhea, possibly reflecting that some of these procedures were more difficult[21].

However, patients' satisfaction, and the occurrence of postoperative pain and rate of re-TCRE and hysterectomy showed no differences. Thus, fibroids without symptoms related to size are not a contraindication for TCRE in patients with bleeding disorders.

Endometrial thickness and uterine size

Preoperative endometrial thickness represents a predictor of postoperative amenorrhea[20]. This is according to the common belief that preoperative pharmacological thinning of the endometrium gives a shorter operation time and improved results[28]. So far, however, controlled studies to support this view are not available.

The preoperative TVS data from the present series[20] also suggested that patients with a small uterus assessed by the anteroposterior diameter had a shorter operation time showing fewer operative difficulties and less glycine deficit. Uterine size and the presence of fibroids that deform the uterine cavity are factors thought to be important regarding the clinical outcome of TCRE. However, no such relationship between uterine morphology assessed by preoperative TVS, the hysteroscopic findings and the therapeutic effect of the procedure could be shown in our present study. In contrast, the endometrial thickness at the time of surgery had a significant impact on the results. Patients with an endometrial thickness of 8 mm or less were more likely to experience amenorrhea. This effect did not relate to the day of the cycle on which the resection was done, as no relationship was found between endometrial histology and either residual endometrium or clinical outcomes. It seems that outcome is dependent on the quantity of endometrial tissue present. These data therefore support the use of agents that induce endometrial atrophy prior to TCRE, such as danazol or gonadotropin releasing hormone analogs. Whether similar results can be achieved if the operation is done during the postmenstrual phase when the endometrium is naturally thinnest remains to be seen. Of further interest was the fact that women with a smaller uterus (anteroposterior diameter < 53 mm) experienced a shorter operation time and less glycine deficit (Table 1). In addition, significantly more patients experienced amenorrhea when the anteroposterior diameter was less than 53 mm; these findings could be related to the fact that the operative procedure was not always complete due to operative difficulties. The mean glycine deficit for women with an anteroposterior diameter of > 53 mm was 809 ml, showing that a large uterus per se, although making the procedure more difficult, is not a contraindication to TCRE.

It is also of interest that the number of patients with residual endometrium detected at TVS increased significantly during the follow-up period, reflecting the regenerative capacity of this tissue. Thus a scan performed too soon after the operative procedure cannot select all those women who have received a suboptimal resection, with perhaps 6 months being the optimum time for follow-up. Residual endometrium may represent viable tissue with a capacity for regeneration. It is, therefore, important to remove even small nests of endometrium left behind between the resection grooves during the procedure. Taken together, the data available show that half, or more, of the patients have significant amounts of residual endometrium despite a satisfactory clinical result after TCRE. The discrepancy between our findings using ultrasound and such histological findings are hardly surprising. TVS can only give an indication as to the likelihood of endometrium being present. In contrast, histological assessment of biopsies from the cavity may detect small microscopic nests of residual endometrial tissue[15]. This is clinically important as hormonal replacement

Table 1 Operative parameters and clinical results in relation to uterus dimensions (means and standard deviations in parentheses)

	Anteroposterior diameter		
	< 53 mm	> 53 mm	p
n	98	77	
Operative time (min)	20 (7.8)	26.6 (12.7)	< 0.05
Glycine deficit (ml)	603 (603)	809 (895)	< 0.05
Bleeding index 12 months	5.9 (10.5)	7.2 (8.8)	NS
Amenorrhea 12 months	64 (66%)	34 (45%)	< 0.05

therapy should clearly be given as combination therapy to avoid the development of endometrial hyperplasia and malignancy in such women. TVS represents an attractive method for further study in the postoperative long-term follow-up of TCRE patients after the menopause, since endometrial thickness may be a helpful parameter in selecting women at increased risk of endometrial malignancy[29]. In another study performed at our center, these issues have been investigated[30] to determine if women who have undergone TCRE can safely be treated with estrogens alone. Sixty-two postmenopausal women who had undergone transcervical resection were recruited to the trial. Patients were allocated to one of two hormone replacement therapy (HRT) regimens (17β-estradiol 2 mg monotherapy group or 17β-estradiol 2 mg combined with norethisterone 1 mg combined therapy group). Clinical and ultrasound data were collected every 3 months. Hysteroscopically standardized endometrial biopsies were taken after 1 year. In the monotherapy group, endometrial hyperplasia without atypia was found in six patients, and proliferative endometrium in eight after 1 year. Endometrial thickness and menstrual bleeding were significantly greater in the monotherapy group compared to the combined therapy. In the cases of hyperplasia, the mean endometrial thickness measured by ultrasound was 11.8 (range 6–16) mm. Hyperplasia was never histologically observed when the endometrial thickness was 4 mm or less. In cases of proliferative endometrium, the corresponding value was 7.4 (range 4–18) mm. Postmenopausal HRT in patients who have undergone TCRE should include progestogen protection of the endometrium.

In our series, an intrauterine fluid collection was found in 13 out of 188 patients; however,

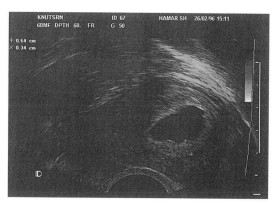

Figure 2 Hematometra after transcervical resection of the endometrium

only six had symptoms of uterine outflow obstruction. In a previous series, hematometra was diagnosed in two of 50 patients 3 months after TCRE[17] (Figure 2). The data therefore suggest that this may occur after TCRE but in itself does not require correction without symptoms.

In conclusion, the presence of some submucous fibroids has no impact on the clinical outcome of TCRE and need not be a consideration when selecting patients for this procedure, although fibroid size may represent a factor worthy of future investigation. The main indicator of the outcome was preoperative endometrial thickness, with an endometrial thickness of less than 8.0 mm being associated with a significant increase in the number of women becoming amenorrheic 1 year following the procedure. By contrast, the day of the menstrual cycle on which the procedure is performed does not seem relevant *per se*. The data support the use of therapeutic agents that may lead to a reduction in endometrial thickness, or to doing transcervical resection of the endometrium in the immediate postmenstrual period when the endometrial thickness is naturally least.

References

1. Rybo, G. (1986). Variation in menstrual blood loss. *Res. Clin. Forums*, **4**, 357–74

2. Rybo, G. (1966). Menstrual blood loss in relation to parity and menstrual pattern. *Acta Obstet. Gynecol. Scand.*, Suppl., **45**, 7

3. Cameron, I. T. (1989). Dysfunctional uterine bleeding. *Baillieres Clin. Obstet. Gynaecol.*, **3**, 315–27

4. Nilsson, L. and Rybo, G. (1971). Treatment of menorrhagia. *Am. J. Obstet. Gynecol.*, **110**, 713–20

5. Coulter, A., Noone, A. and Goldacre, M. (1989). General practitioners' referrals to specialist outpatient clinics. II. Locations of specialist outpatient clinics to which general practitioners refer patients [see comments]. *Br. Med. J.*, **299**, 306–8

6. Long, C. A. and Gast, M. J. (1990). Menorrhagia. *Obstet. Gynecol. Clin. North Am.*, **17**, 343–59

7. Studd, J. W. (1989). Hysterectomy and menorrhagia. *Baillieres Clin. Obstet. Gynaecol.*, **3**, 415–24

8. Dicker, R. C., Scally, M. D., Greenspann, J. R. *et al.* (1982). Hysterectomy among women of reproductive age. Trends in the United States, 1970–1978. *J. Am. Med. Assoc.*, **248**, 323–7

9. Backe, B. and Lilleng, S. (1993). Hysterectomy in Norway. *Tidsskr. Nor. Laegeforen*, **113**, 971–4

10. Loft, A., Andersen, T. F., Bronnum Hansen, H., Roepstorff, C. and Madsen, M. (1991). Early postoperative mortality following hysterectomy. A Danish population based study, 1977–1981 [see comments]. *Br. J. Obstet. Gynaecol.*, **98**, 147–54

11. Dicker, R. C., Greenspann, J. R., Strauss, L. T. *et al.* (1982). Complications of abdominal and vaginal hysterectomy among women of reproductive age in the United States. *Am. J. Obstet. Gynecol.*, **144**, 841–7

12. Langebrekke, A., Eraker, R., Nesheim, B. I., Urnes, A., Busund, B. and Sponland, G. (1996). Abdominal hysterectomy should not be considered as a primary method for uterine removal. *Acta Obstet. Gynecol. Scand.*, Suppl., **75**, 404–7

13. Rankin, G. L. (1995). Safety and transcervical endometrial resection [letter]. *Lancet*, **345**, 56

14. Magos, A. L., Baumann, R., Lockwood, G. M. and Turnbull, A. C. (1991). Experience with the first 250 endometrial resections for menorrhagia [published erratum appears in *Lancet*, **337**(8753), 1362] [see comments]. *Lancet*, **337**, 1074–8

15. Istre, O., Skajaa, K., Holm Nielsen, P. and Forman, A. (1993). The second-look appearance of the uterine cavity after resection of the endometrium. *Gynaecol. Endosc.*, **2**, 189–91

16. Khastgir, G., Mascarenhas, L. J. and Shaxted, E. J. (1993). The role of transvaginal ultrasonography in preoperative case selection and postoperative follow up of endometrial resection. *Br. J. Radiol.*, **66**, 600–4

17. Cornier, E. (1984). The Pipelle: a disposable device for endometrial biopsy. *Am. J. Obstet. Gynecol.*, **148**, 109–10

18. Stovall, T. G., Solomon, S. K. and Ling, F. W. (1989). Endometrial sampling prior to hysterectomy [published erratum appears in *Obstet. Gynecol.*, **74**(1), 105]. *Obstet. Gynecol.*, **73**, 405–9

19. Chimbira, T. H., Anderson, A. B. and Turnbull, A. C. (1980). Relation between measured menstrual blood loss and patient's subjective assessment of loss, duration of bleeding, number of sanitary towels used, uterine weight and endometrial surface area. *Br. J. Obstet. Gynaecol.*, **87**, 603–9

20. Istre, O., Forman, A. and Bourne, T. H. (1996). The relationship between preoperative endometrial thickness, the presence of submucous fibroids and the clinical outcome following transcervical resection of the endometrium. *Ultrasound Obstet. Gynecol.*, **8**, 412–16

21. Istre, O. (1996). Transcervical resection of both endometrium and fibroids: the outcome of 412 operations performed over 5 years. *Acta Obstet. Gynecol. Scand.*, **75**, 567–74

22. Lewinski, H. (1931). Beitrag zur Frage der Adenomiosis. *Zentralbl. Gynakol.*, **55**, 2163–4

23. Kilkku, P., Erkkola, R. and Gronroos, M. (1984). Non-specificity of symptoms related to adenomyosis. A prospective comparative survey. *Acta Obstet. Gynecol. Scand.*, **63**, 229–31

24. Nishida, M. (1991). Relationship between the onset of dysmenorrhea and histologic findings in adenomyosis. *Am. J. Obstet. Gynecol.*, **165**, 229–31

25. Scottish Hysteroscopy Group (1995). A Scottish audit of hysteroscopic surgery for menorrhagia: complications and follow up. *Br. J. Obstet. Gynaecol.*, **102**, 249–54

26. Bird, C., Mcelin, T. and Manalo-Estrella, P. (1972). The elusive adenomyosis of the uterus revised. *Am. J. Obstet. Gynecol.*, **112**, 583–93

27. Townsend, D. E., McCausland, V., McCausland, A., Fields, G. and Kauffman, K. (1993). Post-ablation-tubal sterilization syndrome. *Obstet. Gynecol.*, **82**, 422–4

28. Brooks, P. G., Serden, S. P. and Davos, I. (1991). Hormonal inhibition of the endometrium for resectoscopic endometrial ablation. *Am. J. Obstet. Gynecol.*, **164**, 1601–6

29. Granberg, S., Wikland, M., Karlsson, B., Norstrom, A. and Friberg, L. G. (1991). Endometrial thickness as measured by endovaginal ultrasonography for identifying endometrial abnormality. *Am. J. Obstet. Gynecol.*, **164**, 47–52

30. Istre, O., Holm Nielsen, P., Bourne, T. and Forman, A. (1996). Hormone replacement therapy after transcervical endometrial resection. *Obstet. Gynecol.*, in press

Three-dimensional ultrasound of the endometrium and uterine cavity

15

K. Gruboeck, M. Natucci and D. Jurkovic

INTRODUCTION

Ultrasound plays an important role in the diagnosis and management of many gynecological disorders. The introduction of transvaginal sonography and small portable machines has facilitated widespread use of ultrasound in gynecological outpatient clinics. However, despite continuous technical improvements there are still important limitations in ultrasound diagnosis in gynecology. These include a lack of clear diagnostic criteria for the differentiation between benign and malignant pelvic tumors and difficulties in the diagnosis of endometriosis and pelvic infection[1]. Another important problem is caused by pelvic anatomical relations which severely restrict the movements of the transducer during scan. This results in a very limited number of scanning planes available for examination.

Clinical suspicion of uterine pathology is a common indication for gynecological ultrasound examinations. The uterus is relatively easy to visualize in every patient on both transabdominal and transvaginal scans. Fibroids, which are the most common uterine abnormality, can be detected even if they measure only a few millimeters in size. Suspicion of endometrial pathology and localization of intrauterine contraceptive devices are other frequent indications for scans.

The uterus is typically positioned in the center of the pelvis with its long axis lying perpendicular to the ultrasound beam during transvaginal scan. The examination of the uterus is usually restricted to transverse and longitudinal sections which give an incomplete view of the uterine fundus. For that reason, conventional two-dimensional sonography is not adequate for

the definite diagnosis of congenital fusion defects of the uterus.

Three-dimensional ultrasound has recently been introduced into clinical practice[2,3]. This technique overcomes some of the limitations of two-dimensional sonography mentioned above. The major advantages are the ability to obtain ultrasound sections which are impossible to see on a routine scan and perform accurate volume measurements. In addition, three-dimensional anatomical reconstruction of the organs of interest is possible[4].

In this chapter we will discuss the technique and potential diagnostic value of three-dimensional ultrasound of the uterus.

TECHNIQUE OF THREE-DIMENSIONAL SONOGRAPHY OF THE UTERUS

We have performed all our three-dimensional studies of the uterus using a B-mode scanner which monitors spatial orientation of the images and stores these as a volume set in the memory of a computer (Combison 530 3D Voluson, Kretztechnik, Austria). Conventional two-dimensional B-mode transvaginal ultrasound examination is always completed first. Once the uterine position is identified the uterus is visualized in the longitudinal plane. The ultrasound probe is kept steady and the patient asked to lie still on the examination bed. The volume mode is then switched on. Three-dimensional ultrasound volume is generated by the automatic rotation of the mechanical transducer through 360°. The acquired volume is in the shape of the truncated cone with the depth of 4.3–8.6 cm and the angle $\alpha = 90°$. Using the medium line density the typical acquisition time is around 10 seconds.

The obtained volumes may be analyzed immediately or stored and examined later. Computer-generated, planar-reformatted sections are similar to images obtained by conventional B-mode two-dimensional sonography. They are generated very fast and are the simplest way of looking at three-dimensional volumes. Three perpendicular planes are simultaneously shown on the screen thus enabling easier understanding of uterine anatomy (Figure 1). The number and orientation of reformatted planes is not limited, which provides sections through the uterus which could not be obtained on routine scan. The most useful plane is the transverse section through the whole length of the uterus from the fundus to the cervix. This plane, being perpendicular to the direction of the ultrasound beam spread, cannot be seen on a conventional transvaginal scan.

Volume measurements can also be performed immediately or later using stored ultrasound volumes. Our main interest was the measurement of endometrial volume. Three perpendicular reformatted sections are displayed on the screen and a longitudinal plane is chosen for volume measurements. The other two planes are used to ensure that the whole of the uterine cavity has been included into the measurement. The actual measurement is performed by delineating the whole of the uterine cavity in a number of parallel longitudinal sections 1–2 mm apart. The endometrial volume is then calculated automatically by the in-built computer software program (Figure 2).

Three-dimensional reconstructions of the uterus are also possible using ultrasound volumes. Although three-dimensional images in obstetrics may be of some significance, our experience did not show significant contribution of three-dimensional reconstructions to the diagnostic accuracy in cases of uterine abnormalities. The calculations often take around 10 minutes or more and may be helpful only in patients with unusual and complex congenital or acquired abnormalities of the uterine cavity.

THREE-DIMENSIONAL ULTRASOUND FOR THE ASSESSMENT OF THE UTERINE CAVITY

Congenital uterine anomalies are associated with an increased risk of miscarriage, premature

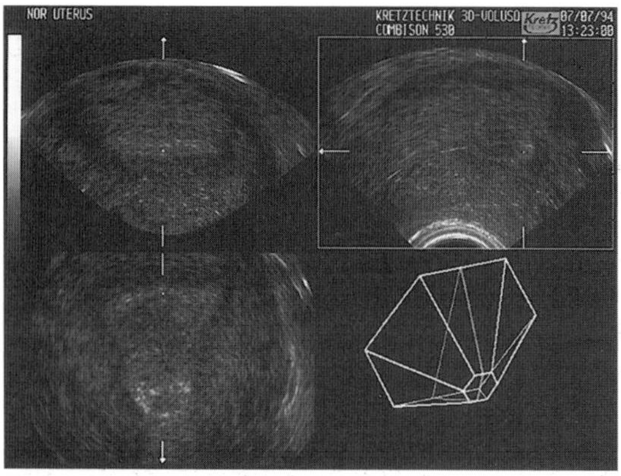

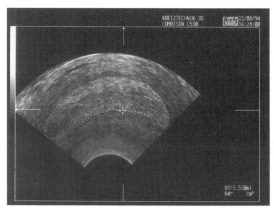

Figure 1 An illustration of three-dimensional volume analysis using planar reformatted sections. Three perpendicular planes are displayed simultaneously. Standard transverse and longitudinal sections of a normal uterus are seen in the upper part of the image. The third section in the left lower corner is perpendicular to the ultrasound beam and for that reason can only be generated by the computer

Figure 2 An illustration of volume measurement using three-dimensional ultrasound. The endometrial area is outlined in a number of parallel sections and the volume is calculated using a built-in software program

birth, fetal loss, malpresentation and Cesarean section[5,6]. The diagnosis of congenital uterine anomaly is usually made in patients with previous pregnancy loss, while the prevalence in the general population is largely unknown. This is partly due to the lack of a simple and accurate diagnostic test which can be used in low-risk patients.

The traditional method for the diagnosis of uterine anomalies is hysterosalpingography (HSG). This is an invasive test which requires the use of contrast and exposure to radiation. Although HSG provides a good outline of the uterine cavity, the distinction between different types of lateral fusion disorders is often impossible[7,8]. In these cases laparoscopy or laparotomy may be necessary to achieve the final diagnosis. Although the recent reports have indicated a high diagnostic accuracy of magnetic resonance imaging (MRI) for the diagnosis of congenital uterine defects[5] the technique remains very expensive, and is rarely used for this indication. Due to limitations of current diagnostic methods the final diagnosis is usually achieved only by combining the results of two or more tests.

Important advantages of ultrasound over other imaging methods are its non-invasiveness, safety and simplicity. Unfortunately, the efforts to characterize congenital uterine anomalies by two-dimensional B-mode ultrasound have not been successful. When used as a screening test transvaginal sonography has provided sensitivity rates of up to 100%[6]. However, the distinction between the different types of anomalies is often impossible[7]. Ultrasound is operator-dependent and hard copy images can be difficult for a third party to interpret. Therefore, other diagnostic methods are usually required to complete the diagnostic evaluation, particularly in patients in whom corrective surgery is planned.

Recently we have conducted a study to investigate whether the additional views of the uterus that can be obtained by reslicing three-dimensional volumes are useful for the diagnosis of congenital uterine defects[9]. Only high-risk patients with a history of recurrent miscarriages or infertility were recruited into the study. They all had a HSG done within 6 months prior to the

scan. The results of HSG or any other previous diagnostic test were not available to the ultrasonographer at the time of the scan.

The American Fertility Society Classification of Müllerian Anomalies[10] was used to describe uterine defects. The criteria for the diagnosis of an arcuate uterus were normal appearance of the cervix and myometrium, absence of fundal cleft and a rounded appearance of the fundal portion of the uterine cavity. In cases of subseptate uterus the proximal part of the uterine cavity was partially divided by a septum. The myometrium appeared normal. However, if a fundal indentation was present it should have been less than 1 cm in depth to allow classification as subseptate uterus. The diagnosis of bicornuate uterus was made when divergent, well-formed cornua were seen separated by a large fundal cleft (> 1 cm).

Good quality three-dimensional volumes were obtained in 95.1% of patients. In 40 out of 44 patients who had normal HSG findings this was confirmed by three-dimensional scans. In all nine patients with arcuate uterus the diagnosis was confirmed by three-dimensional scan (Figure 3). Three patients with major congenital uterine anomalies were also correctly identified on three-dimensional scan. The diagnosis of subseptate uterus was made in two cases (Figure 4) and bicornuate uterus in the remaining one (Figure 5). The presence of large fibroids was also detected in six patients. Three patients with

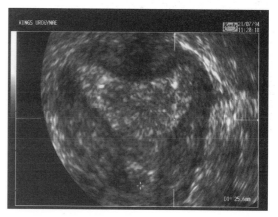

Figure 3 An arcuate uterus on three-dimensional scan shows typical rounded appearance of the uterine fundus

normal uterine cavity on HSG had anterior intramural fibroids which caused shadowing and inadequate three-dimensional images.

Sensitivity, specificity, and positive and negative predictive values of two- and three-dimensional ultrasound for the diagnosis of normal uterus and congenital uterine anomalies were calculated in 58 patients with technically acceptable three-dimensional volumes (Table 1). All cases of congenital anomalies were detected by both two- and three-dimensional scans. Five false-positive diagnoses of arcuate uterus and three of major uterine anomalies decreased specificity and positive predictive value of two-dimensional in comparison to three-dimensional scans. There were no false-positive or false-

negative diagnoses of congenital uterine anomalies with three-dimensional ultrasound[9].

Our results indicate that three-dimensional ultrasound may become an important method for the assessment of the uterine anatomy and the diagnosis of congenital uterine anomalies. In most patients three-dimensional ultrasound has enabled clear visualization of the uterine cavity and the diagnosis of congenital anomalies. The images were easier to obtain in the luteal phase of the cycle due to increased thickness and echogenicity of the endometrium. On examination of stored three-dimensional ultrasound volumes sections through the uterus were obtained within a few seconds. The most useful plane was the transverse section through the whole length of the uterus from the fundus to the cervix. This enabled the measurement of both the depth of the fundal cleft and the length of the uterine septum. This plane, being perpendicular to the direction of the ultrasound beam spread, cannot be seen on a conventional transvaginal scan. This section is also difficult to obtain on transabdominal scans for the full urinary bladder has a tendency to push the uterus backwards with its anterior surface parallel to the abdominal wall. This results in the longest uterine diameter being perpendicular to the ultrasound beam as it is on a transvaginal scan.

Two-dimensional ultrasound detected all cases of anomalies but there were a number of

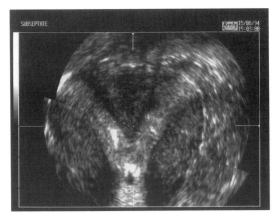

Figure 4 A large uterine septum is clearly demonstrated in a patient with the diagnosis of subseptate uterus

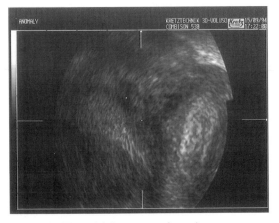

Figure 5 Two widely separated uterine cornua are seen in a patient with bicornuate uterus

Table 1 The diagnostic accuracy of two- (2D) and three-dimensional (3D) ultrasound in comparison to hysterosalpingography in 58 patients with history of recurrent miscarriage or infertility

	Sensitivity (%)	Specificity (%)	PPV (%)	NPV (%)
Normal uterus				
2-D	88	94	97	75
3-D	98	100	100	94
Arcuate uterus				
2-D	67	94	55	88
3-D	100	100	100	100
Major anomaly				
2-D	100	95	50	100
3-D	100	100	100	100

PPV, positive predictive value; NPV, negative predictive value

false-positive findings. The lateral parts of the uterine cavity close to the tubal origin often gave a false impression of an arcuate uterus. In both cases a division of the endometrial echo in the lateral uppermost part of the uterine cavity was seen. However, due to the inability to obtain transverse sections through the long axis of the uterine fundus, the distinction between normal and arcuate uterus is often impossible on conventional B-mode scanning. For the same reason it was hard to differentiate between arcuate, bicornuate and subseptate uteri on a two-dimensional scan. The diagnosis of these anomalies is based on the accurate measurement of the fundal cleft and the length of the septum. These measurements could not be performed on traditional scans and the diagnosis was based on the indirect measurements and a subjective impression of the fundal anatomy. The sensitivity of two-dimensional ultrasound is very high and therefore it can be used as a screening test for congenital uterine anomalies. Three-dimensional ultrasound should be used as a diagnostic test in those with a screen positive result on two-dimensional scan.

Three-dimensional ultrasound for the diagnosis of endometrial carcinoma

Endometrial carcinoma is the most common gynecological malignancy in many developed countries with overall 5-year survival rates of approximately 65%[11]. The reported incidence in women with postmenopausal bleeding is around 10%[12,13]. Therefore invasive tests such as endometrial biopsy or dilatation and curettage are traditionally required to obtain histological diagnosis in all symptomatic patients. Recently, transvaginal ultrasound and the measurement of endometrial thickness has been suggested as a useful test to differentiate between atrophic endometrium and endometrial pathology[14,15]. Endometrial thickness of less than 5 mm on ultrasound was associated with atrophic endometrium on histology in 96% of cases[16]. However, the differentiation between pathological findings such as endometrial hyperplasia and cancer was not possible due to overlap in the endometrial thickness measurements[17].

The volume of primary tumors is an important prognostic parameter in many gynecological and non-gynecological cancers. Until recently it was impossible to measure the volume of endometrial carcinoma preoperatively. Therefore the value of this parameter for the diagnosis, staging and prognosis of endometrial cancer is unknown.

Recently we have used three-dimensional ultrasound to investigate the diagnostic value of volume measurements in patients with endometrial cancer. One hundred and three patients with a history of postmenopausal bleeding were recruited into the study. All patients underwent a transvaginal ultrasound scan using the same three-dimensional ultrasound equipment as described above[18]. The uterus was visualized in the longitudinal plane and endometrial thickness was first measured at the thickest part between the highly reflective interfaces of the endometrial–myometrial junction. This measurement included both layers of the endometrium. The surrounding low amplitude echo layer was not included in measurement as it represents the inner layers of compact and vascular myometrium[19]. If free fluid was present inside the uterine cavity the thickness of each endometrial layer was measured separately and then added together excluding the fluid.

Once B-mode examination had been completed, three-dimensional volumes were recorded as described previously. The endometrial volume was measured by delineating the whole of the uterine cavity in a number of parallel longitudinal sections 1–2 mm apart. The volume was then calculated automatically by the in-built computer software program. The accuracy of volume measurement was checked by using a phantom with a known volume (Unitex Model 50 Phantom, Siel Imaging Ltd, Aldermaston, UK).

Endometrial volume was successfully measured in 97 patients (94.2%). In six patients the presence of anterior uterine wall fibroids caused acoustic shadowing on three-dimensional records resulting in poor images of the uterine cavity. Histology showed atrophic endometrium in 66 patients, normal proliferative endometrium in five, endometrial polyp in seven, hyperplasia in eight and endometrial cancer in 11 patients. Nine patients with the diagnosis of endometrial cancer underwent hysterectomy, bilateral oophorectomy and pelvic lymph node sampling. Two patients were treated by radiotherapy alone.

Endometrial thickness and volume in patients with normal or atrophic endometrium, hyperplasia, polyps and cancer are shown in Figures 6 and 7. In patients with cancer the mean endometrial thickness was 29.5 mm (SD 12.59) and mean volume was 39.0 ml (SD 34.16). The endometrial thickness and volume were both significantly lower in patients with benign pathology. In 71 patients with atrophic or normal endometrium the mean thickness

and volumes were 5.3 mm (SD 3.98) and 0.9 ml (1.72) respectively. This was significantly less than in abnormal cases. Endometrial thickness of less than 5 mm was always associated with atrophic or normal endometrium. However, there was an overlap in the endometrial thickness between benign and malignant pathology. The best cut-off level for the diagnosis of carcinoma was 15 mm which resulted in the sensitivity of 83.3% with specificity of 88.2% and positive predictive value of 54.5%. Endometrial volume in patients with malignant pathology was significantly different from those who had hyperplasia or normal endometrium. With cut-off level of 13 ml the diagnosis of cancer was made with sensitivity of 100%. There was only one false-positive result in a patient with endometrial hyperplasia which gave a specificity of 98.8% and positive predictive value of 91.7%. Comparison of receiver operating characteristic curves for the thickness and volume measurements showed that the latter was more sensitive for the diagnosis of carcinoma at nearly all levels of specificity.

The size of the endometrium was also related to the grade of the tumor. In well-differentiated tumors both the thickness and volume were lower than in moderately or poorly differentiated tumors. In patients who underwent surgery, endometrial thickness and volume were compared with the myometrial invasion and the stage of the cancer. With increasing depth of invasion both endometrial thickness and volume were increased. Comparison of tumor stage and size showed that larger mean endometrial volumes were found in patients with advanced cancers (Table 2).

These results have shown that by using three-dimensional ultrasound equipment it is possible

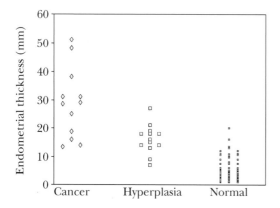

Figure 6 Endometrial thickness in postmenopausal patients with normal and abnormal histological findings. There is considerable overlap in the thickness between different groups

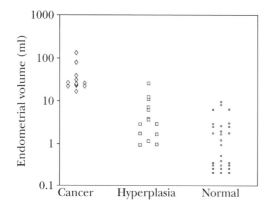

Figure 7 Endometrial volume in the same group of patients. The overlap between the cancer and noncancer patients is minimal

Table 2 Endometrial thickness and volume in relation to the stage of endometrial cancer in nine patients

Stage	n	Thickness (mm), mean (range)	Volume (ml), mean (range)
Ia + b	3	19.3 (13.4–28.5)	23.0 (21.5–24.5)
Ic	3	30.7 (25.0–38.0)	22.0 (13.5–30.0)
IIa	1	48.0 (—)	38.0 (—)
IIIc	2	22.5 (14.0–31.0)	51.5 (26.0–77.1)

to measure endometrial volume in the majority of postmenopausal patients. The measurements are reproducible and more likely to reflect the true endometrial volume than estimations based on the calculation of the volume of an ovoid[20]. The shape of the uterine cavity, particularly in patients with invasive carcinoma, very rarely resembles an ideal ovoid which prevents the use of mathematical formulae for the calculation of its volume. The only way to measure it is to outline its surface in a number of parallel sections which would take into account irregularities of its shape. This is the principle of volume measurement by the three-dimensional ultrasound equipment. The accuracy of this approach has been previously tested in *in vitro* conditions and has proven to be reasonably accurate[21].

Our results also confirm that there is a considerable overlap between endometrial thickness in patients with benign and malignant pathology (Figure 6). When volume measurements were performed the overlap between different groups of patients was much smaller. This has improved the diagnosis of cancer which is illustrated in Figure 7. All but one patient with cancer had large endometrial volumes of more than 20 ml. Using a cut-off level of 13 ml none of the cancers would have been missed but one patient with cystic glandular hyperplasia would have been wrongly diagnosed as positive. Endometrial thickness measurements gave less accurate predictions. In comparison thickness performed best using a cut-off level of 15 mm which gave two false negatives and 11 false positives. False-negative results were eliminated if the cut-off level was reduced to 13 mm. However, this increased the number of false positives to 16.

In patients with very thin atrophic endometrium, volume measurements contributed little to the diagnostic accuracy. When the endometrium looked atrophic with a thickness of less than 5 mm the measurement of endometrial volumes was more difficult. However, all patients with a volume of less than 0.5 ml had endometrial atrophy on histological examination. In patients with endometrial cancer there was a clear tendency for endometrial volume to increase with grade and stage of the tumor. The depth of myometrial invasion showed positive correlation with both endometrial thickness and volume. However, the differences were not large and it is unlikely that the measurement of the tumor size will be more useful for the diagnosis of invasion than B-mode imaging.

Another important finding was a relatively large volume of primary tumors in patients with advanced disease. Only patients with tumor volume larger than 25 ml had evidence of pelvic node involvement at the operation. This result is in agreement with the findings of others who compared the size of endometrial cancer on hysterectomy specimens with the frequency of lymph node metastases. They showed that the risk of lymph node involvement with tumors less than 2 cm in diameter is only 4% and the 5-year survival rate was 98%. The size of the tumor was a significant prognostic factor which was independent of the tumor grade and depth of myometrial invasion[22].

If our preliminary data are confirmed, the volume of the tumor may be used in the future for the preoperative assessment of patients with endometrial cancer. Tumor size combined with other risk factors may improve the selection of patients who require a more aggressive surgical approach, including pelvic and para-aortic lymph node sampling.

References

1. Rottem, S., Timor-Tritsch, I. E. and Thaler, I. (1993). Assessment of pelvic pathology by high frequency transvaginal sonography. In Chervenak, F. A., Isaacson, G. C. and Campbell, S. (eds.) *Ultrasound in Obstetrics and Gynecology*, pp. 1629–41. (Boston: Little, Brown and Company)
2. Jurkovic, D., Jauniaux, E. and Campbell, S. (1994). Three-dimensional ultrasound in

obstetrics and gynecology. In Kurjak, A. and Chervenak, F. A. (eds.) *The Fetus as a Patient*, pp. 135–40. (New York: The Parthenon Publishing Group)

3. Steiner, H., Staudach, A., Spitzer, D. and Schaffer, H. (1994). Three-dimensional ultrasound in obstetrics and gynaecology: technique, possibilities and limitations. *Hum. Reprod.*, **9**, 1773–8

4. Balen, F. G., Allen, C. M., Gardener, J. E., Siddle, N. C. and Lees, W. R. (1993). Three-dimensional reconstruction of ultrasound images of the uterine cavity. *Br. J. Radiol.*, **66**, 588–91

5. Pellerito, J. S., McCarthy, S. M., Doyle, M. B., Glickman, M. G. and DeCherney, A. H. (1992). Diagnosis of uterine anomalies: relative accuracy of MR imaging, endovaginal sonography and hysterosalpingography. *Radiology*, **183**, 795–800

6. Nicolini, U., Bellotti, M., Bonazzi, B., Zamberletti, D. and Candiani, G. B. (1987). Can ultrasound be used to screen uterine malformations? *Fertil. Steril.*, **47**, 89–93

7. Whitehouse, G. H. and Wright, C. H. (1992). Imaging in gynaecology. In Grainger, R. G. and Allison, D. J. (eds.) *Diagnostic Radiology*, pp. 1825–53. (Edinburgh: Churchill Livingstone)

8. Randolph, J. R., Ying, Y. K., Maier, D. B., Schmidt, C. L. and Riddick, D. H. (1986). Comparison of real-time ultrasonography, hysterosalpingography, and laparoscopy/hysteroscopy in the evaluation of uterine abnormalities and tubal patency. *Fertil. Steril.*, **46**, 828–9

9. Gruboeck, K., Jurkovic, D., Lawton, F., Bauer, B., Zosmer, N. and Campbell, S. (1994). Endometrial thickness and volume in patients with postmenopausal bleeding. *Ultrasound Obstet. Gynaecol.*, (suppl.) **5**, 157

10. The American Fertility Society (1988). The American Fertility Society classifications of adnexal adhesions, distal tubal occlusion, tubal occlusion secondary to tubal ligation, tubal pregnancies, mullerian anomalies and intrauterine adhesions. *Fertil. Steril.*, **49**, 944–55

11. FIGO (1988). Annual report of the results of treatment of gynaecological cancer, vol. 20. (Stockholm: International Federation of Gynaecology and Obstetrics)

12. Quinn, M. A., Anderson, M. C. and Coulter, C. A. E. (1992). Malignant disease of the uterus. In: Shaw, R., Soutter, P. and Stanton, S. (eds.) *Gynaecology*, pp. 533–46. (Edinburgh: Churchill Livingstone)

13. Holst, J., Koskela, O. and Von Schoultz, B. (1983). Endometrial findings following curettage in 2018 women according to age and indications. *Ann. Chir. Gynaecol. Fenn.*, **72**, 274–7

14. Goldstein, S. R., Nachtigall, M., Snyder, J. R. and Nachtigall, L. (1990). Endometrial assessment by vaginal ultrasonography before endometrial sampling in patients with postmenopausal bleeding. *Am. J. Obstet. Gynecol.*, **163**, 119–23

15. Osmers, R., Voelksen, M. and Schaue, A. (1990). Vaginosonography for early detection of endometrial carcinoma? *Lancet*, **335**, 1569–71

16. Granberg, S., Wikland, M. and Karlson, B. (1991). Endometrial thickness as measured by endovaginal ultrasonography for identifying endometrial abnormality. *Am. J. Obstet. Gynecol.*, **164**, 47–52

17. Sladkevicius, P., Valentin, L. and Marsal, K. (1994). Endometrial thickness and Doppler velocimetry of the uterine arteries as discriminators of endometrial status in women with postmenopausal bleeding: a comparative study. *Am. J. Obstet. Gynecol.*, **171**, 722–8

18. Jurkovic, D., Geipiel, A., Gruboeck, K., Jauniaux, E., Natucci, M. and Campbell, S. (1995). Three-dimensional ultrasound for the assessment of uterine morphology. *Ultrasound Obstet. Gynaecol.*, **5**, 233–7

19. Fleischer, A. C., Kalemeris, G. and Entman, S. (1986). Sonographic depiction of the endometrium during normal cycles. *Ultrasound Med. Biol.*, **12**, 271–7

20. Shipley, C. F., Smith, S. D. and Dennis, E. J. (1992). Evaluation of pretreatment transvaginal ultrasonography in the management of patients with endometrial carcinoma. *Am. Obstet. Gynecol.*, **167**, 406–12

21. Gilja, O. H., Thune, N., Matre, K., Hausken, T., Odegaard, S. and Berstad, A. (1994). *In vitro* evaluation of three-dimensional ultrasonography in volume estimation of abdominal organs. *Ultrasound Med. Biol.*, **20**, 157–65

22. Schink, J., Rademaker, A., Miller, D. S. and Lurain, J. (1991). Tumour size in endometrial cancer. *Cancer*, **67**, 2791–4

Index